"Every once in a great while, a book comes along that makes us realize the truth in a burst of great joy. *A Practical Guide to Creative Senility* is such a book.

"After you have read it, there are all kinds of things you will never look at in the same way again. The author's light-hearted view of life directs us toward our own humanity and possibilities in a way rivaled only by a combination of Charlie Brown, Lao Tsu, Winnie the Pooh, and a baseball game on a sunny day."

Michael Ray
CO-AUTHOR *Creativity in Business*

This is a novel by Donovan Bess.
The images are by Ruth Eisenhart.

A Practical Guide to Creative Senility

By

Dr. Hiram Podges, Jr.

Blue Dolphin Publishing
1988

Published by Blue Dolphin Publishing, Inc.
P.O. Box 1908
Nevada City, CA 95959

Library of Congress Cataloging-In-Publication Data

Bess, Donovan, 1909-
    A practical guide to creative senility.

    I. Title.
PS3552.E7946P7   1988   813'.54   88-9551
ISBN 0-931892-16-3 (pbk.)

Printed in the United States of America by
Blue Dolphin Press, Inc., Grass Valley, California

9   8   7   6   5   4   3   2   1

Contents

The Formative Years (1907-1976)

The Practical Guide Itself

A Note from the Editor

TWELVE YEARS AGO I WAS studying creative writing at the University of Iowa. I didn't learn much about creative writing, but I did meet Hiram Podges, who was the headwaiter at the faculty club. He was a rosy-cheeked man of sixty-four who liked to stand around near tables where professors were talking so he could listen in. He told me he got a lot of education that way without having to read "thousands of boring books."

I decided to use him as a model for a character in a novella I was writing, and that is how we got acquainted. We would have beers together a couple of times a week. After I moved to Berkeley, he had to quit his job. He got to be worried about getting old. His wife had died a few years earlier. They had been married when he was twenty-six.

One day he wrote me a long letter describing all his woes at being forced to live, as he said, "on the shelf." He thought he was "getting to be senile."

I sent him back my viewpoints. I reminded him, for example, that when retired U.S. Supreme Court Justice Oliver Wendell Holmes Jr. had his ninetieth birthday, President Roosevelt paid him a visit and found him reading Plato and said, "For goodness sake, Mr. Justice, why are you reading Plato?" And the old guy replied, "To improve my mind."

I really loved Hiram. I told him he ought to try to come out West so we could have some more beer drinking together. I was very busy and I'm afraid I neglected our correspondence. But, one day, when Hiram had gotten to be sixty-eight, a nephew of his had moved to Oakland, a city that adjoins Berkeley. This nephew's wife had gotten pregnant, and he invited Hiram to come out and live with them. That way he would get a built-in baby-sitter. He told Hiram the climate in Oakland was fabulous. No more dreary winters in slushy snow, no more summers holed up in the house with iced tea, no more fighting off mosquitoes and bats while on the porch on hot and humid evenings.

I met him at the Oakland train station and we headed for a bar to have a commemorative round of Millers' High Life beer.

He looked older than he had in the Iowa days. But under the new wrinkles there was some very fragile newness. I saw in him a nakedness that could be very vulnerable to the alcoholic push and shove of all the nearby dice-rolling, noisy drinkers; and at the same time he was as rugged as Abe Lincoln.

"Hiram," I said, "it seems to me you look more like yourself now than when you were charge′ d'affaires at the faculty club. What have you been up to?"

There was a half-smile on his face. He looked sideways as though he were consulting a clever, secret friend who knew the answer to my question.

"Pablo," he said, "I don't know what." And he winked at me. It seemed to me that his wink said "I love you," but the "you" was not just me. It was more like the whole world with its ups and downs, its El Salvador death squads as well as its Mother Teresas—its rain and blizzards and its sun that gives us our heat strokes as well as our life.

"All I can say," he said, "is that it was a long tunnel and I came through it and here I am on this end of it."

"What is 'this end,' Hiram?"

He looked down into his mug of beer. He picked it up and held it against the bright sun that was about to set. "All those jewels in there," he said, "they move around constantly and each of them is prettier than any diamond they weigh the Aga Khan with."

"They weighed him with gold," I said.

"They are gold, too—see? And they're on the move constantly. You can't say that about ordinary jewelry."

As we walked out of the bar he grabbed my arm and held it tight. "Listen," he said, "I have seen the power and the glory of senility." His eyes searched my face the way the eyes of an infant carried by its mother into a crowd of strangers pleads for some assurance that it won't be abused by them. "The trouble is," he said, "I've only seen it, and suddenly here's all this California around me, and it's a foreign country, Pablo, and it scares me."

I didn't feel I could find any words for him.

"Yep, all I've done so far is *seen* it. I'm scared that the outside world is mostly against me making it all come true."

I was thinking of Chopin who surely saw "it" and thereafter wrote beautiful music full of the joy of having seen "it" and the melancholy of not being able to reach it.

I knew that Hiram's fragile, new self was going to be tested thoroughly. Indeed, this new Hiram *was* tested by the outside world. From time to time he told me of his adventures and misadventures. Six years later I told him, "You've *really* been creative, Hiram. I try to teach creative writing to college kids and I hardly know what creativity is."

"You know enough," he said.

"Hiram," I said, "why don't you write a book about it?"

He said he couldn't write—"I never even finished high school."

I asked him if he'd be willing to talk it into a tape recorder. I said we could get a student to transcribe it and make it into a book.

"I love that word 'creative'," he said. "That word has to be in the name of the book. And 'senility' has to be in the book, because that's what scares people shitless. It scares them when they get old, and it scares them when they're still young."

" 'Creative Senility'," I said.

"And it has to be *practical*, Pablo. It has to be a guide."

I didn't do much as editor except to tell him now and then when I thought he was rambling too much.

He asserted forcefully that he had become "a genuine expert" on senility, so he wanted to be known as Hiram Podges, Jr., D.S., for "Doctor of Senility."

I argued that this might make people think he was a gerontologist. He said that would be terrible. But I gave into his argument that more people would read the book if the author were called "Dr. Podges."

The cover and the illustrations were done by Ruth Eisenhart, an artist who got herself into the heart of Hiram.

Pablo McGinty

Overture by the Author

SENILITY USED TO BE thought of as a piteous problem. Nowadays, thanks to my personal researches of my own self, plus observations of others, I have learned that your senility can be your road to having a good time right up to the end, not to mention peacefulness.

Although I am only seventy-seven, I began the practice of creative senility about a decade ago. I am only sorry I didn't start sooner. People keep publishing all these guides for how to have sex and how to make money and get fame, but the truth is, if you have good sex and if you make a lot of money and get famous, why would you waste time to write guides about it?

Since I am such a great success with senility, you may well wonder why *I* should take time out to write this guide for you. Listen—I was in Cody's bookstore in Berkeley the other day and all I saw in their old age section were books that treat senility as an enemy. That's not practical!

Authors are supposed to dedicate books. So I hereby dedicate this one to Mr. Pablo McGinty, who inspired me to get off my duff and do it. He is a certified authority on English grammar, proof of which is that he teaches creative writing to the girls at Mills College. He even gives poetry readings! His own poetry!

He showed me how to throw away extra words.

(Signed) _____

Dr. Hiram Podges, Jr.

The Major Characters in this Book

Myself, who did the research on senility that will change millions of life-styles.

Jack Galloway, my nephew, who is trying to become a psychiatrist at the University of California Medical School.

His winsome wife, Margaret, better known as Marge.

Their son Teddy, by now age of six, my really best friend.

Fred Trauerkloss, an old man who lives next door.

His granddaughter, Lillian, a teenage blonde beauty.

Marge's Aunt Jessie.

Various and sundry friends and associates of Jack and Marge, in whose house I am domiciled.

Violet, who was my wife before she died.

Pablo McGinty, who has been like a kid brother to me and corrected my grammar and all that.

My sister, September, mother of Jack, who was sentenced to a "convalescent home" because she failed to make her senility creative, and for this reason is not, after all, a major character.

The Formative Years (1907-1976)

What Sort of Fellow I Am

I GOT BORN IN Cedar Rapids, Iowa, and stayed there for ten years. I was just eleven when I saw my first dead person. Some old guy had flopped down on his back on the sidewalk and I could see by his face that's what death is. All I could think was something like, "That happens to some people and it's *weird*," and I ran off to play softball.

Same way with old folks I'd see here and there—*weird,* like ostriches or giraffes.

I had the standard Iowa Presbyterian upbringing—no problems except that they made me go to Sunday school on Sunday mornings. My dad whipped me a few times and mom wet-kissed me more than I liked, and when the three of us and my sister went to the movies, mom would check my ears when we got to the street car stop and she *always* found they were dirty, so she took out her hanky, spit on it and cleaned them out. That was the worst thing she did to me, so why should I complain? We were like those families by Norman Rockwell that you used to see on the cover of the *Saturday Evening Post* before it went broke—nice, well-scrubbed, happy-go-lucky faces with no big ups and downs.

There were hardly any automobiles around in those days. Only rich people had cars until Ford made his Model T. One afternoon my folks had the honor of being invited by Mr. James Tarlock, the banker, to have a ride in his Marmon. The car got wrecked and both mom and dad got killed.

I was twenty years old, but I admit I shed many a tear for them while alone in my room.

I got married a few years later to Miss Violet Gerber. She was half-Hungarian and half-English. The Hungarian part made her look very mysterious, while the English part made her always ready for a good laugh. We moved to Iowa City so she could attend the University of Iowa, but she only held out for two years. She didn't like all that studying.

When I was fifty-nine, she died on me. That night in the hospital, while I stood by the bed looking at her, I suddenly knew all at once she was *dead*. It was like little hands inside my belly grabbing me tight. She was dead—just as dead as that fellow I saw lying on the sidewalk in Cedar Rapids. But her eyes were wide open, and I saw she kept looking at something. It seemed to me she probably saw that where she was going to was a big, nice surprise, by golly!—even bigger and nicer than, when you're a kid, they bring in the birthday cake with the candles all lit for you to blow out.

I wished I could cry, but all I could feel was amazement at her seeing all that when she was supposed to be dead. After a while some tears came down my cheeks. They were almost tears of being glad for her. I felt sort of uneasy that I wasn't fuller of grief. Then the nurse came in and said, "Hiram, it's all over. I'll just close her eyes." I grabbed that nurse and held her real tight so she couldn't do that. The nurse said, "We *have* to close the eyes." Why should I let the hospital tell me what I had to do about my wife? Other people came in and I was like a tiger and fought them off, and that was how she went to the undertaker, with her eyes seeing something that you and I never can see. Even though they raised me as a Presbyterian, I can't say I was what you'd call religious. But Violet's eyes told me *some*thing, so that ever since then I never was afraid for myself to die. (Well, not all the time, to be honest, but most of the time I wasn't.) For days and days after that, I cried and cried.

Still, I had my position as the headwaiter at the university faculty club. The honor and eminence of my position made me feel I was somebody, and helped me get by without Violet.

Maybe I've wandered off the subject of this book. But you ought to have some idea of what sort of fellow I am.

All the Hard Luck Stuff

GOING IT ALONE IS no picnic. I must have put all of my eggs in one basket—Violet. Weekdays, from 10 to 8 at the club, I got by mainly by concentrating on being extra gracious. I started off with the English "lit." profs. I learned all their names and dished out smiles. I had all of these high and mighty fellows in the cup of my hand, and the time passed fast. I liked the "anthro" folks the best. They study different tribes, such as American Indians and Australian freaks. Their table was right near my station, and I overheard all I could. I learned that our country's point of view, the "American Way of Life," was just one way, not the whole world's, as Mr. Reagan used to claim (except for Russians and Cubans, who, he said, are outside the human race).

I sold our house to get more cash and rented what's called a studio apartment, such as students have. Gee whiz, it was dreary, coming back there at night. The only thing I could cook was boiled eggs, coffee and toast and canned beans.

Fortunately, I had my friend, Per (Pete) Swanson, who also lost his wife, and we played pool a lot. Pete also steered me into a poker crowd that met every Friday night. I watched the TV a lot, but all those advertisements all the time spoiled the shows. Naturally, I indulged in watching *all* the sporting events. I got so I went to watch the Iowa Hawkeyes play in person—basketball, football, baseball and track.

Until I began to move toward age sixty-five, I got by easy. But then things began to happen that really made me wonder. The first time some young fellow called me "sir" I really got a shock.

I always thought of myself as just "Hiram," and suddenly I wondered, was the outside world now seeing me as an old man? Even worse of a shock came when some old friends of Violet and me, the Bergmans, invited me to a Christmas party; their daughter looked right through me as if I was transparent.

Even worse yet, at another party, I was standing in the hallway—all by myself, mind you—when a young beauty waltzed in, and guess what she did? She hitched up her skirt and adjusted her panty hose at the top, just as if I was a cigar-store wooden Indian. I guess I had entertained thoughts that I'd fall in love with some fetching creature who would cry, "Oh, Hiram, I was afraid you'd never ask!" That's the sex part!

As a matter of fact, the night after that happened I went back to my chicken coop and took a hard look in the mirror. Wrinkles and furrows, big pouches under my eyes and, good grief, almost all my hair was gray. I must have known that before but only sort of. This time I had to see what *they* saw.

On top of that I looked at my hands and saw those brown splotches popularly known as liver spots. Undeniable! King Lear in person! When I took a bath I saw all those loose folds where once everything used to be firm and tight. And on the bus, when it was crowded, young fellows would offer me their seats. Sometimes girls would, too, and I *hated* them. And there was nobody I dared talk to about it. I did my best to bury all these ugly facts by doing my job extra well. But at the age of sixty-five they told me I had to quit my job.

That was all I had left, my distinguished service to the professors— and now that was down the drain. I almost went down with it. During that first year of being jobless, I began to get backaches and pains in my elbows, and cramps in my hands. I went to the doctor who said, "You have to expect this sort of thing at your age."

One day I finally went to the library and read up on the subject of senility. I was in line for "progressive hearing loss," absent-mindedness, second childhood, "degenerative diseases," forgetfulness, preoccupation with the years gone by, shrinkage of body size, "incontinence," and "confusion." I could see that what they had in mind for me was to end up in a wheelchair, staring glassy-eyed with a bib around my neck to catch the slobber.

I have always been a fellow who says of a bad situation, "I can lick it." Now the whole wide world was telling me, "We gotcha!"

The next couple of months were the bottom of the barrel. It was freezing cold outside, too. It's a wonder I didn't slit my throat. There's a saying that "hope springs eternal in the human breast." I guess I must have been hanging onto that hope like a man at the bottom of a cliff that somebody threw a rope to.

When the month of April came along and the trees were full of buds and the birds were singing the Hallelujah Chorus, all I could think was "Shit!"

A letter came in the mail. It was from Pablo McGinty in California. He wanted to know why I hadn't answered the letter he wrote at Christmas time. How the hell was I, anyway?

It's funny that when I'd needed somebody to tell my troubles to I should forget those times of beer drinking with him, and how he used to be just as interested in me as I was in him. Funny that I should forget how much I trusted him. In spite of his young age, he knew a lot of stuff I didn't, and he always treated me as if I knew a lot more than I let on to.

"Write me!" he cried in his letter.

And at the end of the letter he said, "Hiram, I really miss you." Heart-warming. Nevertheless, I did wonder if I could trust him far enough to tell him all my miseries.

I finally decided I just had to try it, just let him know it. I wrote it all, all the hard-luck stuff I told you about. Then I got afraid to mail the letter. Maybe he'd changed a lot and would be disgusted with me. Maybe he only liked me when I was cheerful. I stood by the mailbox a long while, fidgeting. But I just couldn't afford to keep this crap to myself one second longer. I just had to drop it into the mailbox, and I did so.

I Get To Be the Prince

THE DAYS WENT BY like years, while I rushed to the mailbox each morning looking for Pablo's verdict. After six days finally went past, I wondered if I no longer had him as a friend. We had met in the era before he became a published poet, before he got his full-time girl-friend, before he got into the famous, glamorous life of California. It is a known fact that friends *can* just fall away at the swish of a horse's tail. I thought of good old Ed Cerruti, my pal when I served in the great war against Hitler. I served merely as a corporal stationed in the godforsaken town of Bruning, Nebraska, where the only vegetation in sight was cornfields. Ed and I spent thousands of hours together playing backgammon or blackjack or going out to bars and getting drunk. What we had especially in common was the weird fact that we both stayed loyal to our wives. The other GI's razzed the hell out of us for that.

We read each other the passionate letters the wives sent us, and sympathized with each other and felt proud of all that devotion from our womenfolk. Another thing we had in common was baseball fever—although I rooted for the Chicago Cubs and he had his money on the Brooklyn Dodgers. Ed came from Missouri, so after the war we'd each take buses so as to meet in Chicago and talk about the good old days in the Army. It looked like our friendship would go on till death did us part. But the whole thing just wore out like an old Ford.

So, remembering that, and while I heard no word from Pablo, I thought to myself, "After all, he's half my age and full of piss and vinegar, so maybe he has no time left any more for this poor old rotting apple."

I was *very sorry* for myself—a full-blown tragic figure. But it was all from my imagination! For, indeed, only eight days had gone by when I got a big fat letter from Pablo.

He told me I should get out of Iowa and come West. He told me, "Flow with your senility instead of fighting it." He said fighting it makes it a disease, but that it actually offers a "real creative potential." "People just don't let themselves get the fun out of their second childhood," he said.

Well, you must admit that these were pretty outlandish ideas. But I admired him so much, I tried real hard to figure out what he meant. I wrote him and told him I respected his ideas but I just couldn't figure them out. He wrote me back saying, "The one way *not* to understand your senility is to try to figure it out. The only way is to be exactly what it is, moment after moment."

And then one night in June I was lying in bed wondering why he kept on telling me these things, and I started to fall asleep. But I didn't really fall asleep. I was in between. I saw a real bright, colored picture of Pablo laughing. That faded away and I saw myself as a little kid, maybe seven years old, throwing a lit firecracker at a horse *right in sight of my dad watching*. I was doing what *they* say a kid must never do—and I felt as high and mighty as Emperor Hirohito of Japan. Then that scene faded away and I saw myself, Hiram, my own self, looking really free of all the opinions in the world, a *prince,* handsome beyond belief, and the prince never remembered he'd been born and wasn't sure he was going to die. He wasn't me at *all,* but he was nevertheless more absolutely, perfectly me than I had ever been. He wasn't a kid, but he wasn't old, either. Then there was a whole big crowd around him yelling and jeering at him. I knew I never could make the crowd see how perfect and handsome I was.

I woke up out of this in-between situation. It wasn't a dream, so it had to be real. Really real.

How the Red Carpet
Got To Be Rolled Out

ONE DAY A COUPLE OF YEARS AGO, while I was listening to the psychology profs at the faculty club, I heard a fellow talk about a theory from Switzerland. The theory was that outside events sometimes seem to follow the lead of something that's happened in a person's head.

"Sheer, mystical poppycock!" one of the profs cried, with big emotion. The whole psych table broke into laughter. It was obvious they had ruled that the theory was farfetched.

I remembered that theory the day after the night that I realized I was Hiram the Prince. I remembered it because two days later the outside world rolled out the red carpet for the prince.

How this carpet got rolled out has a lot to do with what families are. I mean, a family has a mom and dad and from one to twenty offspring, plus maybe a grandma or grandpa thrown in. According to the rule of fate, some of these folks can be saints, while others are as mean as all

14

get-out. The family you're born into is like the dice roll in a game of craps. In my case, the dice rolled out mom and dad—good luck. They also rolled out my two sisters. My big sister, Emma Lee, I found out, was bad luck.

When Emma Lee was a kid, she picked on me so I tried to stay clear of her. On Saturday night, which was bath night, Emma Lee and I had to sit in the tub together so as to save on hot water. She *always* made me sit in the back of the tub so she could have the warm water up in the front.

But I figured that when she grew up we could forget all that kid stuff. Alas, no! She married a Swede named Bjorn E. Swanson. He was a major general in the Salvation Army and he had a stiff little moustache, and never did I see a smile bloom beneath it.

As the years rolled by, Emma Lee got so she looked just about the same as that famous lady in a painting called "American Gothic." In this painting the lady stands alongside a gent who's obviously been her husband for decades. He is holding a make-hay pitchfork. You can see that both of them are absolutely sure that they know what is right, and that anybody who argues with them will end up dead wrong. A couple of years ago Emma Lee "passed on to her reward," as the saying goes. If there's a Hereafter, I'm sure she's busy telling St. Peter how to redecorate it.

Then there is my little sister. My mom gave her the name of September on grounds that that month was the nicest one of the year.

She always was and she remains the sweetest of the sweet, and she always looked up to me.

September married James Galloway, a professor of Bible at Macalester College, a Presbyterian school in St. Paul, Minnesota. That sounds bad. But, fortunately, he was what they called a "liberal." For example, he believed that the story of Jonah being swallowed by the whale was merely a way of saying that if a fellow really trusts the Lord, he can be swallowed that way and will be better off for staying a while in a whale and for experiencing the deep sea in a way that ordinary folks never get to have.

September and Jimmy both had a habit of laughing a lot, so Violet and I would take any excuse to visit them. We were always welcomed with open arms. They had three kids. Violet and I never could have kids, so it was always a big treat to go up to St. Paul and see what this new generation was up to.

September and Jimmy's youngest kid, the boy, was Jack. He and I got to be very chummy by the time he was nine years old. Their family had a summer cottage on Lake Minnetonka. Violet and I were up there for a while every summer except when I had to serve some time in the Army.

I was Jack's favorite uncle. I taught him how to swim and how to fish. One July day in a boat, he caught a pickerel that measured to fourteen inches. It was a mighty proud moment for him when September served up what he'd dragged out of the lake. He dearly loved the different trees and animals of Minnesota, and we'd take long hikes together.

Violet and I also spent every Christmas up in St. Paul in their house on St. Claire Avenue. The best gift I gave Jack was a Gilbert's chemical set. He passionately loved to fool around mixing different powders in liquids and seeing all the mysterious changes. I also gave him his first toboggan, which is a kind of sled, that he took to the toboggan slide in the woods next to Macalester College. They poured water on the slide so it became ice and you'd ride down that slide at a hundred miles per hour.

When Jack went to Central High School, he got to be wild about science, especially biology. He ended up majoring in pre-med. When he was nineteen, he met a girl from California, name of Marge, who was visiting her aunt in St. Paul. He fell in love with her at first sight. She was the reason he decided to try to go to the University of California Medical School in San Francisco. Jack saved quite a sum of money doing construction work summertimes. His dad and I also pitched in so he could pay for this big project in San Francisco. Jack and Marge got married.

As you can see, my mind wanders. That is one of the best advantages of senility—they don't expect you to stick to the point. All this wandering was to help explain how come I ended up in California. It has a lot to do with the theory those psych. profs were joking about—the theory that sometimes when a fellow gets a certain frame of mind inside his head, things happen outside that are sort of the outside equivalent of the inside idea. I told you about the visions that showed me I really was the prince. The visions came after Pablo argued that I oughtn't try to *figure out* how my senility could be creative. Those visions just flew in on me in the night. It was only two days later that this letter from Jack comes saying Marge was eight months pregnant and I would be most welcome to go out and live with them in Oakland, California. They said they had a guest room that they would sign over to me. I was Uncle Hiram and I'd also be their built-in baby-sitter.

I figured I could learn how to change a diaper so that the safety pins don't get stuck in the baby.

Broken Promises!

BACK IN IOWA it's plenty easy to make up a picture of California as the Promised Land. I knew there were big mountains and palm trees and Chinatowns and the ocean, which I'd never seen before. No wonder so many folks deserted Iowa to go out West.

I hate airplanes. I found out there was a train that went from Chicago to Oakland. I wanted to know by personal experience what those two thousand miles were between us and California.

Golly, what a huge country the U.S.A. is! First there was a corner of Iowa and then Nebraska—flat miles forever and ever over country I knew from Army days to be godforsaken. I sure did wonder why the invaders from back East hadn't just let the Indians keep it.

Our train finally made it uphill into Colorado and there were millions of tall pine trees outside. After Denver we had to cross Wyoming—which was pretty, and then across Utah, and then across Nevada, which was as forlorn as the moon.

Reno, Nevada, the famous divorce city, turned out to be real pretty, and suddenly we were across the border into California. There were millions of even bigger pine trees than in Colorado and snowbanks as high as the State capitol building in Minnesota. Then we went downhill and ended up in a big valley full of freeways on which millions of cars and trucks rushed here and there. I asked the conductor where were the famous orange trees, and he said I'd have to go four hundred miles south to find the oranges and the beaches and the famous movie stars.

Broken promises!

The train got in three hours late. I phoned Jack. His wife, Marge, said he had to be at a conference "in the City" (which I found out means San Francisco), but that Pablo would come pick me up. I felt like a wet dishrag waiting there in that chilly railroad station. It was a great joy when at last I saw him hustling toward me, smiling. He took my suitcases and hustled me into his 1964 Volvo car. He drove us to a bar.

"This calls for a commemorative beer session!" he cried.

Pablo delivered me to Jack's house, which was located on a slope above Lake Merritt. As I found out, how you rate in Oakland depends on your altitude. If you're a rich lawyer or banker, you live high up in the hills where in the forests you can peek at San Francisco across the bay—a pretty sight as long as you don't go over there and mix into all that mad rush. If you're poor, like most of the Negroes, you live in the flatlands. Jack, on his slope, lived amid folks not very rich and not very poor.

Marge laid out the polite welcome mat for me. Her stomach was so immense I thought the kid would pop out any minute.

When Jack got home I guess he forgot how he always used to hug dear old Uncle Hiram. "Welcome," he said, and he shook my hand. And he frowned. "You look really different," he said. By that he meant I looked *old*. He hadn't seen me since I was age sixty-three, which was just before I began to get senile.

Privately, I stuck to the discovery that I was Hiram, the prince—but I guess people judge you a lot by your body looks. I had to conclude that for Jack and Marge the prince was invisible. At supper Jack told me how much fun he had trying to become a psychiatrist at the medical school in the City. But he and Marge treated me as if I was a visiting dignitary.

When I was in bed that night, I knew that my creative senility might come upon hard times in the Promised Land. As the weeks went by, I realized that even more. I found out that California is a country full of desperate people who moved West to escape the cruel climate back East. They have their dreams of Paradise shattered. Millions of them jump off the Golden Gate Bridge.

Most everybody in California has a scheme for how to get more rich or how to get more muscles or how to be more sexy or more famous or how to find Salvation. I guess that keeps the wolf from the door. Trouble arrives, however, if, as in my case, some of these fellows decide their scheme is just the ticket for me.

By the time 1984 rolled in, I had achieved the age of seventy-seven. Pablo and I conferred about my book and I played him the tapes of what you've read (I hope) so far.

"Too much foreplay," he declared. "You have to get them into the *practical guide.* You've told *me* of the joys of forgetfulness. Tell the public, too."

"I have trouble remembering it all."

"And the joys of second childhood," he said, "and your investigations of mind wandering as an art form, and the tests the psychologist gave you, and all that about how to survive those who would kill you with kindness, and the horrors of a visit to the doctor, and—"

"It's all coming back to me," I confessed.

"Not to mention your raptures, such as your perfect friendship with Teddy, and—"

"Yes!" I cried, "Oh, yes!"

Pablo is a leading authority on grammar and has poems published in the *Risen Phoenix* (he said that's a bird that flies up out of an ash pile), so who am I to argue with him.

"I can hardly wait to get into the practical part!" I cried. We clicked our mugs of Miller's High Life beer in a toast to that.

The Practical Guide Itself

Forgetfulness,
the Finest Flower of Them All

IT TOOK A WHILE FOR ME to get settled in at Jack and Marge's. I got my own TV set, and when April came I used the back porch a lot, just sitting in the sun. And I began to explore outside. I especially liked taking the bus to the University of California in Berkeley, where there were 30,000 students and, of these, 5,000 were awfully good-looking girls. Marge was a good cook so I loved eating with them, although Jack seemed to have gotten the notion that I was on the skids. I especially loved Marge's pineapple upside-down cake and her Virginia spoonbread served with baked ham.

I hate to admit this, but I was aghast at the idea of having a baby pollute our cozy little home. When they brought Teddy home from the hospital, he looked to me like a mistake, but when Marge put him in the bassinet I could see he might have a potential to be a human being. As the weeks went by, I confess, I didn't care for all that bawling in the middle of the night and his puking in his pinafore and being constantly wet. Still, one time when the phone rang, Marge shoved him into my arms and a real nice juice flowed up my arm from the warm little bottom of this fellow who was just starting out. As more weeks went by,

I couldn't help notice how fast he was turning from being a blob into a real creature. For instance, when I put my finger in front of his eyes, he looked at it completely. I mean, his seeing the finger was not separated from the finger just being a finger. He was getting all the dope he needed to know about what a finger is, not by trying to figure out what it was.

Just wait till you're senile, and you'll see you too can let go of all the adultness that makes the world stale. It was my being senile that set me free to start to get into Teddy's world. *That* is friendship. How many grown-ups do you see doing it with each other? (Violet and I did sometimes, but we couldn't make it last. Sometimes with Pablo, too.)

After a few months I found out that Teddy was a full-fledged Teddy. That's why I had to shudder as I watched Marge and her friends goo-goo at him as if he was some sort of dumb zoo monkey.

On the first day that he mastered the art of crawling, he crawled all the way into my room (to show me, I bet). What a grin! I watched him a lot during the next couple months, and I knew he was not in any particular hurry to start walking. Crawling was perfect!

During those first years in Oakland my researches into senility got up a mighty head of steam. One thing I observed was that people think retirement equals bidding adieu to life. I told Pablo about this. The dictionary, he declared, gives five definitions of retirement. One definition is "to retreat in battle." He said that is the definition the masses use. I said a better way to look at it was that to retire was to put on a new set of tires.

The public thinks you're only alive and kicking if you work at a job—you go somewhere you don't want to go and do things you really don't want to do. In Iowa City I had to set the alarm clock in order to get up, thereby cutting off the best part of my sleep five mornings of the week.

These days, if I get up early, which is almost never, my heart goes out to those piteous folk rushing downtown or over to the City, rushing wildly to jobs that will only give them backaches and headaches or worse. Before sundown I see the same crowd racing back from work and limping exhausted into their homes, to be revived by adoring wives and a few stiff drinks. (Although in this new era I must say it is frequently the wife who limps home exhausted to fall into the loving lap of the husband.)

Jerry Perlman, who lives across the street from us, is only fifty years of age, I'd say, but he looks like a hundred when he staggers into the house after a day of working as a bookkeeper for some fellow who is paid well to make sure nobody in the office will relax for one minute. Jerry is so used to being a slave, he doesn't know what to do on weekends except watch TV sports, drink gallons of beer, and mow the lawn. In fact, he constantly worries that when he has to quit his job, fifteen years from now, his life will be in ruins.

Jerry works from nine till five in San Francisco. Each morning he races out of the house holding some toast he didn't have time to finish and runs desperately for the bus; and if the sun is gloriously shining, he doesn't even have a chance to notice.

Jerry told me it is the custom in San Francisco for all the toilers in the Financial District to rush into bars after work and guzzle drinks for an hour, so they won't have to spend the rush hour lined up on freeways behind other cars and being almost suffocated by the carbon monoxide, not to mention the boredom. They are pretty plastered by the time they reach the wife and kids, so when the missus asks, "How was your day?" they have to have another two drinks to keep themselves from beating their wives.

After dinner they try to enjoy a little TV, but they are so exhausted the only thing to do is to have sex, which fortunately does provide the one thing in the day that makes it worth living.

After five days of slavery, the weekend comes to Jerry, and on the weekend he's as much out of it as King Tut is. You have to be a slave for years and years to prove you're a loyal American. If you stop doing it, they'll claim you have "retreated in battle."

I do admit there were a couple of times when I worked at the faculty club that I talked myself into believing I enjoyed overhearing the high and mighty blarney broadcast by the professors, but the truth is, I made myself enjoy it to keep from slitting my throat.

When I arrived in Oakland I expected the public would congratulate me on my getting out of my job the way that they congratulate people like Attorney General Mitchell and Vice President Agnew when they get out of prison. I really did. But what I always got was the question, wherever I went, "Are you retired?" They use that word like they've just fished it out of the privy. They made me feel so guilty saying "yes" that I just started telling them, instead, that I no longer have an employer ordering me when to get up, what to do all day and when to go to bed at night. Some of them come back with, "Oh, you are self-employed." I'm supposed to be doing something *useful* or I'm not patriotic.

There'd be no use telling them I can have a heck of a good time just sitting around the house or on the porch not even reading or listening to the hi-fi. No use to tell them about my frequent outings to the Berkeley University campus, which are a real treat. Once or twice a week I take the Telegraph Avenue bus to Stuart Street so as to walk to the Campanile, the campus watchtower. En route I check out the coeds on the street, and the guitar music and the flower stands, pushing my way through the throngs of long-haired, unshaved fellows who ask you for spare change. I pause at Sproul Plaza so as to hear some anarchist make a speech to the jeering brain-trusters or I watch some white-faced clown do amazing juggling. There are card tables where very nice poeple ask you to sign their petitions—"Save Cuba," "Abolish Congress," "Down With Housewives!" I sign all their petitions.

The other day Pablo told me about an Irish myth where a village ran out of water. They sent a guy down the road toward the well. A horribly ugly old lady blocked his path. "No water," she said, "unless ye kiss me." The guy fled in horror. Another guy was sent along this path: same result. A third one came, and he said, "Not only will I kiss thee— I'll give thee a hug." The witch turned into a beautiful young princess who welcomed him to go get water. She told him his name was "The King of No Matter What."

Well, there's a store in Berkeley that sells T-shirts and you can put your own motto on them. I got a scarlet T-shirt and had put on it "I'm the King of No Matter What." I wore it proudly. But putting stuff on a T-shirt is allowed only for persons under age 30. A young guy said to me, "Just what kind of a King are you trying to be, anyway?" Of course, the women in Marge's coffee klatch were upset. "Some of the girls," said Marge, "feel that it's very inappropriate for you to wear T-shirts, and also that mottoes on T-shirts and bright red garments are bad form in one's mature years."

Naturally, I bought myself a bright yellow beret to match.

Speaking of "retired folks," Maitland Viets dropped by to see me. His nickname is Matey. He and his wife moved out of Iowa City to sunny Los Angeles. He said he had to quit his job as cashier at the faculty club because they thought he got too old. The way he talked, you'd never guess he'd ever really managed to get out of Iowa.

We had a few beers together and he comes in with stuff like, "Remember the time Harvey Golden's boy dove off the river bridge even after the police dared him not to? What a ruckus that set off!" Haw, haw, goes Matey. I told him my mind was a blank insofar as the whole Golden family.

"Golden?" I said. "I don't remember any Goldens in Iowa City."

"He was in our senior class play," cried Matey. "His dad was our Scout master."

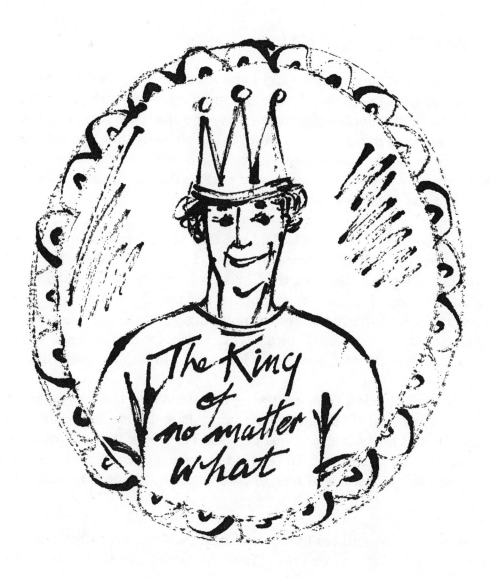

"Well, I'll be darned," said I.

I started telling him about sights he should see in the Bay Area, such as the trees in Marin County that grow sideways instead of up and down, and the Exploratorium in the City, and the cable cars, and the crookedest street in the world, and all the other stuff that tourists from Iowa love so dearly. But Matey bounced back with two dozen more "Remember . . ." stories—every shred of it stuff I had thrown away years ago and hoped was safely down the drain.

It's all over and done with! And not only is it done with for me, but for everybody who lived in Iowa City then. It doesn't exist anymore, no more than the games between the Christians and the lions in the stadium in Rome. I tried, nice and polite, to wedge into Matey's constant soliloquy the idea that he might enjoy letting go of all that dead crap. His retort was that good old Iowa City did exist for him and was in fact even more vivid than whatever was happening to him in California.

"Hiram," he cried, "you are trying to tell me that the best years of our lives do not exist!" He gave me a funny look. I have been getting looks like that lately from various persons. It's a look that sort of says my brain is not up to snuff. To be a red-blooded citizen I should load up my brain with thousands of tons of stuff that's not happening any more.

Matey stood up all red-faced and I could see our friendship was on shaky ground. "Listen," he cried, "these memories are all we have. They are so very precious to those of us who have lived our lives."

"I'm still living mine," I said.

The simple truth is that of all the things that attracted me to creative senility, forgetfulness is first and foremost. It is the finest flower of them all, I sometimes think.

I first saw the light—only a little bit at first—at a party the Bergmans gave. That was when I was still in Iowa City. Some strange fellow showed up and I got introduced. A couple of days later I ran into him by accident at the grocery store—and darned if I could remember his name. I worked and worked at it. I knew the first name was Dave and the last name, I figured, had to do with a color. I scrunched up my face trying to remember. Was it Brown? Was it Blue? Green? Next I decided it had more to do with a house. Newhouse? Nope. I tried combining a color with a house. Greenhouse?

I got in a panic. Was I getting *senile*? At that time I had the same idea most people had, that catching senility was worse than catching syphilis, and I would disgrace the whole family.

Praise the Lord, it flashed into my head—what is wrong with my forgetting the name of some fellow who wasn't even my friend and never would be. Why should I waste all that time fishing for a name I had no use for? When you're over sixty, every five minutes gets to be worth a whole day, so why waste it? I got to wondering about the enormous pile of stuff that had been stored up in my brain. It struck me that most of it was useless junk. I experimented—I shut my eyes and watched the stuff go by, mile after mile, like on a tape.

One item that drifted by was the party they gave me in Iowa City when I had to quit my job at the faculty club. Champagne and a painting of me head-waiting, and the "he's a jolly good fellow" song. My chest swelled with importance and my favorite waitress was even weeping. I saw that it was a movie I had run a lot, and that it was now ten years out of date, grade B, so what's the point of re-running it? I mentioned this to Pablo and he said being creative was not to let the brain cut me off from whatever was happening right this instant.

Champagne that has been drunk ten years ago can't hold a candle to champagne that's on the table right now in the house.

I decided I'd just work on remembering what mattered. For instance, in the supermarket you'll never catch me forgetting the name of Joneses' little pork sausages because I'm wild about them and eat them over and over again. You'll never hear me say Smith's little pork sausages or Brown's little pork sausages.

(P.S. I finally did remember the name of that guy in Iowa was not Greenhouse, but Barnhill. And what in the heck did that do for me, anyway?)

I am a Guinea Pig

I CONFESS I WAS DISAPPOINTED that Jack the grown-up had begun to put on airs—as a result, I reckon, of mixing with all those high-powered brains at the medical school. He had grown himself a beard and whenever we met, which was usually at the dinner table, it seemed to me that he looked at me as if I was a specimen to study instead of good old Uncle Hiram. I am pretty good at overhearing and one day while in my room I heard Jack tell Marge, "You know, my observations about Hiram are giving me some ideas that I might want to revise my career goals." I overheard him telling Marge that in the year 2020 most people in the U.S. of A. will be over age sixty-five. He said there were only three hundred geriatricians in the whole country and there was a big future for geriatricians. Marge asked him what was a geriatrician and he said, "Like a pediatrician, except it's for second childhood. You get similar symptoms in both first and second childhood, such as being inappropriately spontaneous." He said the "real kids" are out of it because they're afraid of the future, but the second-childhood ones are out of it because they're afraid of "their coming demise." You notice he said "demise" instead of "death." He was not even thirty years of age and he behaved as if his lifetime would never end. Lots of folks behave that way, even some old ones, like William Saroyan, the famous author. I read in the paper that when he got so sick it was obvious he was about to check out, he told a friend, "I always knew everybody has to die, but I always thought I would be the exception."

Whenever Jack tackles a project, it runs away with him. Such enthusiasm is admirable for his career purposes. As the months rolled by and he got more and more into being a geriatrician, I became more and more a handy object of experimenting. One night at about 10 p.m., he asked me what was the meal I ate last—breakfast, lunch or dinner.

"It was just before I turned in last night," I said. "Two chocolate-chip cookies Marge bought at the Cookie Magoo's which she forgot to hide from Teddy and me, and also a glass of half and half." Jack smiled at me the kindly way he smiles at Teddy. A snack is not a meal, he said. I asked him why anybody should care what name a meal has. I said what was important was what you ate and how good it tasted.

He put his arm around me. "It's a game, Hiram," he said. "Just for the fun of it, tell me the name of the meal you had this morning."

"Grape Nuts with whipped cream and brown sugar and what was left of Marge's mushroom omelette. I don't like eggs much, but I took it so as not to hurt her feelings."

He has gotten to using a notebook lately when we converse, and he went into his bedroom and got it and wrote in it. "What was the name of that meal you ate, along with the coffee?" he asked. I replied that the meal changes every day so there can't be just one name to cover it—"like yesterday it was Rice Krispies and bacon, but no coffee because we ran out of coffee."

It seemed to me he looked a little bit irritated. He said for me to forget about what I ate and just to tell him what name society has given to the customary American morning meal, "whether it be with eggs or not, with or without coffee." I said that for high society it would probably be a French word, but for us it probably would be an American word.

As a lad I was an apprentice printer, so I can read upside-down type. I saw that he had written in his notebook "random amnesia." I guess that means careless forgetting. As soon as I saw *that* I said, "Oh, Jack, I know that the morning meal is called breakfast, but what if it's not a sincere meal, like Marge yesterday only had half a cup of coffee with a tiny glass of orange juice?" He closed his notebook. I said, "Who won the game, Jack?"

"It's a tie," he said, and patted me fondly on the back.

They Try to Coop Up

IN THE SOUTH they used to have doorways "for whites only" or doorways "for Negroes." Nowadays if you get old enough to be considered out of it, they try to coop you up in "senior citizen centers." Did you ever hear of a junior citizens center?

They probably got the idea from corporations that get rid of an ornery fellow by making him a vice president. The public gets rid of old people by giving them the honorable, highfalutin title of "senior citizen"—they try to keep them out of sight. Or else they call you "elderly"—but never "old."

If you're a kid you're just a kid, and after a while you graduate into being a youth, and somewhere between being age thirty and sixty-five they don't give you any label because with all the hair dyes and the face-lifts and stuffed bras, middle-age doesn't exist. Did you ever really believe that Ronald Reagan didn't secretly dye his hair black?

My friend Lillian came by the other day with her boyfriend, Al, in tow. I must have already told you she is the blonde beauty who comes over on Thursday nights for help with her geometry. "Al," she says, "may I present Mr. Hiram Podges, my geometry tutor."

I could see that I was being shown to him as a remarkable-for-your-age specimen. His handshake almost crushed my hand.

"I hear you attend the A's games," says Al. "That's a real long trip from here."

"I survive it," I said.

"Al," says Lillian, "is the first-string guard on our school basketball team. He was written up in the *Tribune*."

"Did you go in for sports in your day?" he asked.

"The farthest I went was croquet, unless you count canoe paddling," I said.

"Hiram really tries to keep up," said Lillian. "He goes over to the Cal campus a lot. He even works out on those muscle machines at the Courthouse Club."

"Great," cries Al. "That's really just terrific!"

"I was voted the Bay Area senior citizen of the month," I said.

"No kidding!" exclaimed Al.

"He *is* kidding," Lillian declared.

Kids like Al think they're going to live forever.

I knew I'd made it into senior citizen land one night about ten years ago, back in Iowa. I was heading for a cafeteria line at the same time that a young fellow was. We were neck and neck. Suddenly he bows out of the race and says to me, "Go ahead, sir." Little old me is now a sir!

As I mentioned, young dames looked at me as if I was made of cello-wrap. But out here in Oakland I gradually began to think I had wasted a lot of time feeling important just because some dame eyed me. When you come down to it, it was just my body that they eyed, and the body is just temporary housing.

The truth is, Violet and I had all the sex I need for ten lifetimes. For all those years we did every possible combination. I admit I still like to eye ladies. But (if you'll excuse the expression) horniness can get you sidetracked. When I think of the days before I got married, taking girls out in the canoe on the Iowa River, I was so horny I hardly noticed I was on a river and how green and nice-smelling everything was, and the pinkness and the smell of the wild roses on the river banks, and the sounds of frog croaks and the fish jumps.

I still have lustful feelings, but the difference is that these days I just stare at the horniness, and I can see very plainly that it would only bring me more complications than I can use. I shared these thoughts with Marge. "Oh," she declared, "I think it's marvelous that you're not turning into one of those dirty old men."

That night in my room I took off my TV earphones and heard Marge repeating to Jack what I had been telling her.

"The poor guy can't get it up any more, that's all," Jack said. "My heart goes out to him."

The truth is I "get it up" often enough. Actually it gets itself up—you can't train it the way you train a dog, to sit or lie down, or to do tricks.

My mind seems to have wandered away from the topic of senior citizenship. My mind wandering is very precious to me. Pablo wanted me to have a whole chapter on *Mind Wandering as an Art Form*. Let me say, however, that as a senior citizen, I don't mind getting equal financial status along with small children and military personnel. I go to the best movies for two dollars. The barber charges me only four-fifty for cutting what hair is left. On the rapid transit trains I go to San Francisco for only eighteen cents. And at the cheese store, fifteen percent off!

But don't ever admit that you're an *old man*. I went to a movie theater the other day and I asked the ticket fellow did I get an old man discount. Dirty language! "We have a senior citizen discount," he said, holding his chin up high, "if that's what you want." They can't stand to think of anybody as old. Even the government's study committees call us "the aging." Don't they know that every darned kid in our block is aging, not to mention every palm tree and every hook-worm. Indeed, the entire California shoreline is surely but slowly disappearing. So is the city of Venice, Italy. And where do you think our planet is going to be in a few million years?

I Live on the Goal Line

DURING MY FIRST YEAR at Jack and Marge's, Marge was a little bit aloof with me. Maybe she was afraid she'd soon have a basket-case on her hands. But during my second year there, she loosened up a lot. It seemed like part of her—a small part—detected that the longer I lived the more good I got out of my senility. By the way, did I mention to you that Marge is a *looker*?

She has dark-red hair that she lets fall to the bottom of her neck and she is, if you'll pardon the expression, *stacked*. I am proud to say that I have managed not to have one horny thought about her. If I had any such a thought, our home life would go down in ruins.

Sometimes she tells me things she'd never tell an outsider, such as how she regrets that she didn't become a fashion model instead of a mere housewife. I must say, though, that she acts kind of cool towards me when Eloise comes over. She is a gal Marge met at a weekend workshop on *The Alchemy of Flower Arrangement*.

Eloise lives in Silicon Valley, where everybody makes $100,000 a year inventing new-fangled electronic doodad's for the American public to play with. When she came over the other day, she was wearing her designer jeans and gold bracelets and earrings and bright red shoes with high heels. Marge very graciously invited me to share some blueberry muffins and tea with them. I am wild about her blueberry muffins and would gladly eat them with the Hottentots.

"How is life for you, Hiram?" Eloise asks, "now that you're retired?" When she smiles it makes creases in her face like you see in patent leather party shoes. What she really was asking was, "Now that you've lived your life, how bad is it?"

I did not disclose to her the hardships I went through before Pablo wrote me that historic letter that resulted in my discovery of the fact that I was a prince reveling in my senility.

"It was a joyous day when I chucked my job in Iowa City," I declared, "and no longer had to worry about whether the waitresses gave the professors enough to eat and drink."

"I can see you are contented," said Eloise, "but there must be underlying sadness for you in the winter of your life."

"Winter?" I said. "It doesn't seem a bit chilly to me, and I get my hair cut for $1 off, not to mention a discount at the movies, and. . . ."

"What is the goal of life for you, now that you are a senior citizen?"

"Goal? I always live on the goal line, Eloise. The goal right now is to taste the marvelous bluebells Marge put in these delicious buns."

"They are *not* bluebells," Marge said, frowning, "they're blueberries."

"Call them what you will," I declared, "for me they ring like Sunday church bells in my stomach. The goal is chewing them. The goal this very morning was going to the U.C. campus where thousands of comely coeds daily charm the visiting wanderer."

Marge winked at Eloise. That meant I was an adorable oldster. "What is the purpose for you, then?" said Eloise.

Purpose? The truth is, even when I was a callow youth I never stopped to ask what life was supposed to be for. Before I could make up an answer for Eloise, Marge told her, "Hiram has made a wonderful adjustment to his retirement."

I told them, "I always think of adjustment as having to do with carburetors."

We had run clean out of muffins and it was a sunny day, so I retired (excuse the expression) to the back porch where I have my wicker chair and can enjoy dwelling nowhere but where I happen to be.

Marge and Eloise are convinced that my hearing isn't too good. I didn't mind listening in on them. "At least," said Marge, "he never complains and that's a comfort." Eloise retorted, "Remember George Perry's dad? He went totally senile only two years after the bank forced him into retirement."

I was real proud the way Marge rushed to my defense. "Hiram's been retired for seven years," she said, "and he's still not a full-blown senile case."

"That remark about carburetors," said Eloise, "that's not normal. You're too close to him to notice the deterioration."

Oftentimes, when I have my back-porch siestas in the sun, it is my custom to unzip the top part of my pants zipper so as to give the lower part of me more air. Sometimes I forget to zip it back up. It was unzipped on that day, as I walked through the dining room towards the front door. I told them I was going to hike down to Lake Merritt, which is something I frequently do, to enjoy watching the mothers trying to corral their kids and the joggers about to drop from exhaustion as they do their manly laps around the lake.

Eloise slapped her fingers against her lips and cried, "Oh, my!" She was staring, aghast, at my pants. It is a sin for an old man to allow his fly to be even part open. Maybe *they* think you're not supposed to have a pecker any more, or that it's not right for it to be in good working order.

"*Please,*" cried Marge, looking with piteous eyes at the hole in my pants. She comes from a Presbyterian family, and Eloise was a

Methodist. They had paper napkins on the table with pictures of blue ducks on them. I took one of their pretty napkins and stuffed it into the hole in my fly. The ladies were blushing too fiercely to talk. I smiled at them as I walked to the door.

I'm sure Marge told Jack about the zipper catastrophe—and that doubtless inspired him to give me another of his famous senility tests. He came into my room after dinner with his notebook and sat down. Here is how our talk went:

Jack: Hiram, what day is this?

Me: What do you mean by "what day?"

Jack: Like is it Monday the 12th or Sunday the 8th?

Me: Monday is wash day and I didn't see any washing around here today.

Jack: Is it Sunday?

Me: Everybody knows that on Sunday the kids go to Sunday school and the grown-ups sleep late in hopes of wearing out their hangovers. I didn't see anything like that today.

Jack: Hiram, old boy, you're stalling.

Me: All right, let's say it's Tuesday.

Jack: You're getting warm.

Me: Wednesday.

Jack: Wonderful! Right on the button!

I guess he forgot he was supposed to be studying my senility—he was rooting for me to win the game. After all, his mother was my sister.

"Now that I have discovered it's Wednesday," I said, "give me a high score. But does that make it a better day than if it was called Thursday or Friday?"

"What matters," he said, "is our being aware of the world around us. Today, I'm told, you went out with your fly open and a napkin stuck in there."

"Jack," said I, "I knew a fellow who could tell you the batting average of every Dodger player since 1961. Now, I love baseball, but let me tell you that despite my enormous admiration for the Oakland A's, I don't know anything about them except what I see at the ballpark. Seeing Rickey Henderson stealing home is something I absolutely will not consider forgetting—it can be used over and over again. I never remember my own birthday until they bring in all the gifts and sing their song. I used to remember Violet's wedding anniversary because if I didn't all hell would break loose, but I sure don't need to drag it up today, now that she's been underground all these years."

Jack let out a big sigh. I could see I wasn't scoring high. "I *never* remember my dentist's appointment," I said. "Why should I? I even blank out where his office is. If I remembered everything that happened during my sixty-nine years in Iowa, including some side trips to Chicago, my mind would look like Stinson's Beach after a Hell's Angel barbecue."

He shut his notebook, said goodnight and left.

I got to musing on how well I remember exactly when Lillian is due to come over for her geometry lesson. She is the comely granddaughter of Fred Trauerkloss next door. She comes over at 7:30 p.m. each Thursday night. Do you think I could possibly forget on a Thursday morning that come nighttime she will come into my room, wearing her sawed-off Levi's, her beat-up tennis shoes and other items dear to the young ladies of this era? Not to mention the goodnight hug at 8:30 p.m.

Come to think of it, I didn't bury Violet. She was cremated.

Killing with Kindness

ONE THING THAT SENILE PEOPLE do is to attract certain people who specialize in being kind. I have nothing against kindness, but it can go too far.

Marge's Aunt Jessie is one of those people. When I first moved in here I'd see Aunt Jessie jawing with Marge and hardly noticing me even when I was right smack in front of her at the lunch table. But one afternoon when she arrived, she brought with her a bunch of Sweet William flowers. "I've been thinking about you, dear," she said. "I don't want you to feel out of it."

Aunt Jessie was, I would say, fifty-five years of age. She was very vigorous in her getup. At the time, she had orange hair, but when I first met her she had light-brown hair. I've heard her tell Marge a hundred times how everybody keeps telling her how well-preserved she is and how everybody keeps asking, "however in the world do you do it?"

I thanked her for the Sweet Williams and asked her what was the "it" in a person's "feeling out of it." She gave me a big grin. "I'm so glad you asked me that question, dear," she declared. (When they start calling you "dear" that means they think they can help you *cope*. According to the dictionary, "cope" means "to be a match for." Am I supposed to be in a wrestling match with my senility?)

She got a chair and sat close to me. "It," she said, "is the whole vast pulsating world that beckons to us even when we get old and weary and downhearted."

"If it means the world that Jack reads about in *Time* magazine," I said, "I am very glad to be out of it—all those murders and foul play and political mudslinging."

She patted my leg as if I was a little kid. "You won't find 'it' in the magazines, that's true," she said. "As Robert Browning once said, 'God's in His heaven, all's right with the world.' We tend to forget that, don't we, in the sunset years." She looked at my face as if trying to solve a puzzle. "You are not really out of it, Hiram, I can see that. You just *think* you are out of it, dear. You are only as old as you think you are."

There came into my mind the day, a few years ago in Iowa just after they made me quit my job, while in the bathtub, when I found a gray hair growing in my private parts and with great horror plucked it out. I didn't think up the idea of growing that hair gray, nor to make the liver spots that adorn my hands. I got used to these telltale signs of old age but finally found out they won't kill me.

51

"I'm exactly as old as I am," I said. "Nonetheless, there's a part of me that's just like Teddy. Is Teddy out of it, too?" (Teddy at this time was pretty near to three years of age.)

She gave me a smile that was like the smile a nurse gives a patient that's about to breathe his last breath.

It got so that Aunt Jessie brought me flowers almost every time she came over. (Flowers, as everyone knows, are the standard way of extending sympathy to someone gravely ill. The more flowers you get, the nearer you are to death's door.)

After each time she brought me flowers, I rushed to the bathroom mirror to see how much deterioration had set in. When I sat on the back porch, each blossom in the garden told me "the end is near."

The last time she brought flowers they were red carnations. "A little something to brighten up your room, Hiram," she said, patting me on the back. "Red" she declared, "stands for life. On Mother's Day the men wear red carnations to church if their mothers are alive, and white carnations if their mothers have gone on to their reward. Inhale deeply, dear, and take in the life-giving vibrations of the red."

I took the carnations into the kitchen and put them into the wooden bowl Marge uses for chopping stuff for salads. Aunt Jessie watched as I got out the chopper and started chopping up the flowers.

That was the last time she brought me flowers.

They Think I'll Lose My Balls

LET ME OBSERVE, at this point, that although it's not too popular to say it these days, the truth is that the male is different from the female. There are two ways of being kind to old people—the female way, like Aunt Jessie's, and the male way. The males think senility will make a fellow lose his balls.

Such a fellow is Lew Sodhunter. He's a friend of Marge. She met him at a workshop on *The Tao of Jogging*. He wrote a book called *Fitness and Middle Age*.

Workshops are a favorite pastime for California folks. They get high on the weekend and stay high until Wednesday, when they sign up for another workshop. Lew also leads workshops—the latest one is on *The Baseball Diamond Sutra*. He gave me a leaflet advertising it. The leaflet says "through sport we connect you with the beautiful diamond you really are." He also wrote a how-to-do-it sex book. He wears his hair in black bangs. He grins a lot.

Well, he caught me taking a nap in my wicker chair. "Hi, Hiram!" he cried, and he slapped his hands together the way Mr. Dickerson our high school football coach used to when he was exhorting us to get out there and fight for the old school. He asked me, "Feeling kind of down, old boy?" His question made me feel kind of down. "I read the answer in your face," Lew said, "and I know just how it is—you think the whole world is passing you by. Hiram, you've just got to hang right in there with 'em right to the end. Don't *ever* give up!" He danced his body around the way a prize fighter does and he jabbed the air with his fists. "Think of Jean Borotra," he said.

"Who's he?" said I.

"The immortal Wimbledon champion!" he cried. "When he was eighty-seven he played three matches in a tennis tournament. Think big!"

"Well!" He did his big hand-clap again. "We'll start off with a little psychological workout."

He gave me a very serious look. "Close your eyes," he commanded. It seemed like the wisest thing to do was to graciously yield. I shut my eyes. He asked me what did I see. "I see farmers going around with huge bins of candied sweet potatoes and leaving them on people's front steps," I replied. "In the distance the Campfire Girls are singing, 'Oh, Rose Marie, I love you'."

"Very positive images," Lew said, "Now let it get dark and see just one image—let it be a human male image. All right? Nod when you see it." The image came fast and I nodded.

"All right, all right!" he cried, "Beautiful! Now describe what it is that you see there, Hiram."

"What I see is a handsome young Chicano hops picker in a gold uniform. He has just gotten married and he sits on a bright red saddle astride a black panther. He is holding a huge yellow chrysanthemum and he grins at me."

"Look closely, Hiram," said Lew. "Does this man stay young? Do gray hairs show up? Do wrinkles appear in his face?"

"Nothing like that," I said.

Lew folded his arms and frowned. "The image you see is supposed to be a mirror image," he said. "It's not supposed to be some romantic playboy."

I confessed to him that all my life I had trouble seeing the things I was supposed to see. "It has gotten me into a lot of trouble," I said. "That's why I could hardly finish high school—they give you too many supposed-to's."

I asked him how he thought up the game. He said a "holistic psychiatrist" taught it to him. I said I'd like to play another round. I shut my eyes and saw that the handsome young man had taken his seat on a throne and a crowd of fetching young ladies sat on the carpet in front of him, just the way they do with gurus. Lew asked if the image had changed. "Same young hero," I said, "only now he's being admired by some ladies."

"I *see*," he said. "The reality is that as the years roll by, one is drawn more and more toward living in fantasy. What we need to do now is lay a solid physical foundation—and the fantasies will just vanish. Poof!

"It so happens, my boy, that I have at home some instructions for morning exercises specifically designed for the senior citizen. I'll bring over the Pal-Relax Bar, so you can hang upside down for a while when you first get up in the morning. The fantasies go into the feet, where they become harmless. I can get you a Pal-Relax Bar wholesale. I'll also bring over the Ma Roller. You lie with it under your back and before long your stimulated spine seizes the contents of the brain and you're free of all your worst fears. I'll also bring instructions for your diet. I'll show you how to make your seaweed smoothies—and other dietary aids. The kelp and mushroom soup is my favorite for lunch."

I looked at him with what probably was a rather bleak expression. He leaned over so his face was very close to mine. "Pablo Picasso," he said, "was screwing at the age of ninety. So was Henry Miller. So was George Bernard Shaw, the renowned vegetarian author. And Charlie Chaplin. You can be just like them!"

I said I wouldn't mind being like them but that I would prefer not to hang upside down from the Pal-Relax Bar.

"You're resisting," he said. He snapped his fingers at me. "Hiram," he cried, "what are your feelings right now, in this very instant? Don't think—give me what pops into your head."

"The same as usual after lunch," I said. "Almost always I have my nap on the back porch and enjoy being all alone with the sun on my face not having to do anything."

"Hiram!" he cried, "buck up! You're good for another ten years! Today is the first day of the rest of your life. Do you have a girlfriend?"

Since the age of one I have been known far and wide as having what mom called "a good disposition." That means that I avoid arguments and try to think positively as recommended by the *Reader's Digest*. Therefore it is rarely that I think of somebody as a pain in the ass.

It was therefore a surprise to me that I had gotten to feeling that Lew Sodhunter pretty much was a pain in the ass.

"Yeah," I said, "I have a girlfriend."

"Fantastic!" he exclaimed.

"Her name is Lillian," I said. "She's a teenager. She lives right next door. Blonde, really *built*. She comes over to see me every Thursday night." Lew was frowning. "I am quite fit," I said, bowing low toward my privates. "Sometimes, indeed, Lillian sits in my lap. In fact. . . ."

"Hiram!" cried Lew. His chin was quivering and he jammed his lips together tight. "Please do not give me the details."

Lew did not bring over the setting-up exercises or the Pal-Relax Bar or the Ma Roller or the instructions for the diet. Whenever he came over with Jack, as a matter of fact, he did not converse with me. Indeed, he declined even to look me in the eye.

When I related to Pablo the adventures Lew Sodhunter tried to get me into, he just laughed. It is always a treat to pass some time with Pablo. Unfortunately, he lives way up in the redwoods in a cottage on a hill above the Cal football stadium and he has his girlfriend there and gives poetry readings and is busy as a bee, so I never go bother him unless I'm kind of desperate. What he told me about Lew was, "He's afraid *he'll* get senile and not enjoy it as much as you do. Isn't that why you're going to do your book, to educate the masses about the creativity in senility?"

Bright Red Means Keep Out

JACK AND MARGE pestered me for five years to go get a medical checkup. Jack even got emotional about it one night when he had too many of his Tanqueray martinis. "Hiram," he says, putting his arm around me, "it would really bother me a lot if you had some terrible disease eating away at one of your vital organs." I thanked him for his interest, but I just had to remind him that I was like the Model T we had back in Iowa—when she needed a tune-up, she let you know, loud.

After telling him that, he gave such a piteous look that I gave in, and I went to see the doc—who could not wait to ask me did I ever forget where the house I live in is. Gee whiz! How could a person forget anything that important?

Strangely enough something happened a couple days after I saw the doc that made me think a part of me even *wanted* to forget that. The incident was that instead of going to bed in my bedroom, I found myself heading toward the bed in Jack and Marge's room, and I wondered why my bed looked so big. What I encountered was two happy skinny-dippers very busy at America's favorite indoor sport. Marge pulled the sheet up over her bare bosom and screamed to high heaven. Jack looked like a bass that has just been caught.

Jack carried his coffee into my room the next morning for a man-to-man talk. "Hiram," he said, swallowing his Adam's apple, "about last night."

Me: What about it?

Jack: You know, the, uh, that is, your coming in.

Me: Maybe I treaded heavily, for I had indulged in a few beers too many over at the Tail o' the Cock.

Jack: You don't remember coming into our room?

Me: Why should I go into your room, Jack? I got all I need in my room.

Jack put his cup of coffee on the table and covered his face with his hands. His distress moved me so much that I said, "Actually, Jack, I guess maybe I might have strayed into your room. You don't have anything to be ashamed of."

Jack was blushing red as a ripe persimmon. He looked about eight years old. He swallowed hard and said, "What Marge and I are going to do is paint the door of our room bright red. Bright red means keep out. Right?"

Right.

"And we will paint the door of your room bright green. Right?"

Right.

Suddenly he grabs me hard by the shoulder. "Please listen carefully," he pleaded. "We want to live here together harmoniously, so there must be strict rules of behavior. The system we are going to use is the same one used in traffic lights, red for stop and green for go. Now what does bright red mean, Hiram?" I said it meant not to barge in on naked people even if they are part of your own family. That *really* brought on the blushes.

"And what does bright green mean, Hiram?"

"It means," I said, "that all is well in the world. Green is the color of the buds coming out when springtime starts. It is also the color of summertime lawns that invite you to lie on them except when it's raining."

"Yes, and green also invites you to lie down in your own bed, Hiram. Now listen. We'll paint a bright green line on the floor right up to your door. One line will come from the dining room and the other line will come from the kitchen, because that's where you have your bedtime chocolate. When you go to bed, Hiram, please *follow that line*."

"Sure," I said. "I was thinking anyway that the house is a little drab. There's only one thing, though, Jack, which maybe I never got around to telling you about." His face lit up with boyish eagerness to hear what I maybe never told him. "The trouble," I said, "is that I'm color-blind."

"You mean you see red when it's green and. . . ."

"Yes, Jack. At Christmastime I get the colors backward. The truth is I almost got killed hundreds of times after they put in those traffic lights in Iowa City."

Teddy was standing in the doorway. "I want a line for *my* room!" he cried. "I want a zigzag line."

"Why aren't you in nursery school?" Jack cried. Teddy disappeared. But his idea stayed behind. Jack said it could be a straight line to my room and a zigzag line to Jack and Marge's. I argued that Teddy had dibs on the zigzag. Jack graciously agreed to a straight line for me, a wiggly line for Jack and Marge, and Teddy's line zigzag.

When Lillian came over for her next lesson, she asked how come all the lines on the floor. I recounted for her all of the drama just as I told it to you. "At my age," I declared passionately, "if you forget something, they think you're on the verge of throwing in the towel."

Lillian is not as dumb as she looks. She told me that great men who have important ideas forget the things that don't need to be remembered. She said that Albert Einstein, the famous physicist, got the habit of walking right past his house, so his wife painted the door a bright color so as to get him into the right house. Me and Einstein, buddies!

A Self-made Basket Case

NOW IS A GOOD TIME to tell you of the sad plight of Lillian's grandfather, Fred Trauerkloss. Although he is only sixty-six, he walks around bent over like he's looking for trash to pick up. He lives mostly in bed or he's on the back porch if the weather is perfect beyond belief. When he manages to lift an arm to scratch his scrawny neck, you'd think he had a hundred-pound weight on it.

It was only five years ago that Fred and I together built the redwood fence that separates his backyard from mine. He retired from his job as a railroad dispatcher just a year ago. His sixty-fifth birthday was a ceremony to tell the world it was just about all over for poor Fred. Ever since then, if there was any hard luck to be found, he rounded it up.

I've tried to keep being his friend through this downhill slide. A couple of months ago I talked him into having a beer with me despite his argument that it would bring on a case of colitis, whatever that is. The beer ignited a spark in his eyes and he recalled with joy the days when as a lad he played as leftfielder on a Class A farm team of the Boston Braves. Aha, thought I, now I'll have a pal to go with me to the Oakland Coliseum and root for the A's. No such luck. "I would try to go with you," he said, "but I cannot face having to see all those husky young athletes running around in such good shape."

When I go visit Fred his topics are as follows:

1. His arthritis.

2. The fact that all the old friends are "dropping like flies every day."

3. The tragedy of his having to empty his bladder three times each night.

4. His fear of getting cancer.

5. The absence of his wife, Louella (deceased 1975).

6. The deep sorrow that he missed all those chances to make the money that would have allowed him to have a home in the hills with an octagonal swimming pool with cabanas.

7. He worries that he's "turning into a parsnip."

8. The constant headaches, stomachaches and assorted fancy back pains that go along with the above-mentioned items.

9. He's overwhelmed with the sorrow of losing the immense piles of strength, power and virile glory that flowered in what he called "the best years of my life."

"You know what, Hiram," he declared, "I used to be able to lift Herb (his son) with one arm when he weighed a hundred pounds. Now look at me!" He then proceeded to give me an inventory of all of the achievements of his younger days. He groaned as though in dire pain and cried, "All that gone, Hiram, never to return again!"

When I visit Fred I try to turn his thoughts into the positive channels recommended in the classic books of Norman Vincent Peale, the evangelist. For instance, I reminded him how lucky he was that Lillian so often fondles his bald pate and is the model loving granddaughter.

"She is kind to me," he said, "because I have one foot in the grave." I mention how much Lillian has done for our block by planting tons of sweet peas and petunias and watering them constantly. "She is a good Christian girl," he declares, "and not a night goes by that I don't wake up in a cold sweat from worrying that somebody might get her, uh, uh. . . ."

Me: Pregnant?

Fred (hanging his head): Yes.

Me: Did you ever ask her does she go out with boys?

Fred: She has this boyfriend, the basketball hotshot.

Me: Did you ever ask her did she sleep with him?

Fred: I should say not, Hiram! It would kill me if she said she did.

I forgot to mention he also is afflicted with insomnia. I advised him that when I'm not sleepy at night I turn on the light and read *Redbook* magazine, which is not interesting enough to keep me awake.

Fred: At this stage of my life I can't concentrate on reading. The eyesight.

Me: I saw you reading the *Tribune* this morning.

Fred: I only read the one page, the obituaries. I have to find out if there are any of the old friends left.

Me: Those death notices are printed in very tiny type.

Fred: If I squint I can make out the names.

He simply does not get any good out of his senility—he promptly launched into an eloquent complaint about his arthritis. Cruel, cruel pain! And the other day he advised me, "My hearing is about to go, at last." I just had to remind him how he constantly complains about the loud rock music the kid across the street plays on his hi-fi. I told Fred if he got a hearing aid the noise would be unbearable.

The last time he brought up the topic of his night-peeing problem I told him I'd read in Marge's herbs book that when a person gets old he can cut down on his peeing by eating raw parsley just before hitting the hay. "Alas," says Fred, "I can't digest raw vegetables anymore."

Every morning when he's in the tub, he says, he feels his body all over for the bumps that will prove he's caught cancer. "It could be," he said, "that it's got to my liver. When I check in the mirror, I see little yellow specks in my eyeballs that never used to be there."

And then the tragedy of no money. If only he had invested in Ampex stock back in the fifties, he would be rich. "With just a little foresight," he cried, "I'd have a hundred grand today and I would not be this terrible burden for Herb and Nancy (Herb's wife)."

And now, the famous parsnip topic. With all the propaganda these days for vegetables, endearingly known as veggies, why would anybody not want to be one? There's even a Chinese veggie place in Berkeley, although everybody knows the Chinese are famous for preferring pig meat.

Me: Why is it a parsnip you're afraid of becoming?

Fred: They're yellow—pale, gaunt yellow—and they're tasteless. And what's worse, they have wrinkles.

Me: Why don't you pick a curvy, cheerful vegetable like the tomato?

Fred: You kidding? In my time we used to call a pretty dame a tomato. That would remind me of my lost youth.

I finally decided that trying to argue Fred out of his piteous condition by talking was a waste of effort. So I proposed a game of checkers. I'm pretty good at checkers, but I wouldn't mind letting him win a couple of times—"as therapy" (which is the California word for trying to help some poor critter).

Fred: I never liked checkers.

Me: What game do you like best?

Fred: I used to be good at blackjack.

Me: I'll go over and get the cards.

Fred: Hiram, I'm just not up to adding the numbers anymore.

Silence.

Me: Hey, we could set up a horseshoe court down there in the yard.

Fred (wincing in pain): Hiram, I *told* you about the arthritis.

Me: You said it was mostly in your neck.

Fred: It's spreading fast.

Doctors Think You Are Statistics

To TELL THE TRUTH, Fred Trauerkloss is one of the main inspirations for this book. One of his main problems is that he goes and sees doctors until his money runs out. One week it's the internist, next the urologist, next the neurologist. From my own personal researches into myself I can tell you this: if you're old, *don't go to the doctor.*

A pal I met in Oakland, Michael Zane, caught cancer of the lung and was chalked up as having one chance in twenty to survive for five years. Poor Mike, sad case, everybody said with a big sigh.

They took his lung out and afterward he had to go see the doc once a month for an X-ray, and the doc always felt around his neck and in his armpits, looking for woeful developments. He came home a piteous, doomed statistic. However his wife, Darlene, and his kid, a college kid, did not treat him as if he was about to drop dead. Every month the battle waged on—the medics cheering for the statistics and the wife and kid cheering for Mike to keep going.

Darlene is quite the California lady. During the sixties she was a hippie. She has been known to snort marijuana on occasion. She kept this secret from Mike, who believed marijuana would rot your brain. One day when Mike limped into the house after being mentally beaten up at the hospital, she soothed him with some brownies just out of the oven. It is quite the rage in California for ex-hippies to spice their brownies with marijuana. After Mike ate only one brownie, his spirits bubbled up so high he reached out for a second helping. Darlene leaped into his lap and lavished him with kisses to prevent his tackling another brownie, which doubtless would have put him into a coma.

What Mike told me later on was that while sitting there with Darlene in his lap he saw a vision. He is an electrical engineer, so visions are not part of his normal circuitry. What he saw in his vision, he said, was "this white light moving in on me and then it was blue, bluer than a bluebird, and it seemed to have a personal center but it was not able to talk, but it gave me a message anyway, a commanding message, namely, that I was the one in charge of my getting cured."

There is a great distance between the philosophy of an electrical engineer dead sober and an electrical engineer whose body has turned into happy waves. "Darling," he told Darlene, "you have inspired me." As Mike rode the waves, he found himself on a tall tower making a broadcast to all of the white blood cells in his body, advising them to notice that the cancer cells were enemies even though they pretended to be innocent bystanders. "Cells!" he cried, "let us not all go down together; let us rise in triumph together."

Such flowery speech making was a whole new style for Mike. Don't belittle it—that was four years ago and Mike today is as healthy as Teddy's Boston bull pup.

You can bet your boots no doctor would prescribe a broadcast cure like that. Here is an example for you.

A while back Lillian got her grandfather (Fred) to come over and have a look at our famous begonia plant. There was some medic visiting Jack and when we introduced Fred to the doc, the doc said "How do you do." That is not really meant to be a question you take seriously. But Fred is very canny in finding openings for his hard luck. "I'm not doing at all well lately, doctor," said Fred. The doc said "Oh?" and turned his back so as to talk with Jack. "It's my left elbow, doc," said Fred, "unceasing pain day and night." The doctor told him he should get it X-rayed. "I did," Fred declared, "and the radiation man said a sixty-six-year-old elbow was bound to have an ache or two."

I happen to know that Fred's right elbow does not ache and it is also sixty-six years of age.

My own personal rule of thumb is: Never go see a doctor unless you get run over by a truck.

I think I already mentioned that Jack and I had a go-around about me getting a medical checkup. Jack said he could not have peace of mind if he didn't have proof I was not sick.

"Hiram," he said, "can you tell me exactly what the condition of your liver is right now? And your prostate gland? And your heart?" He really looked sad. All this time Teddy was running his tricycle back and forth and around us. Suddenly Teddy grabs my pants leg and says, "Grampa, go do what daddy says." I sure did not want *Teddy* to worry about my health, so I agreed to go get the checkup.

Jack's doctor's name is J. Latham Fimright, M.D. He proved to be very good at asking questions, even when he was feeling me over. He put a glove on and rammed his finger five miles up my rear end.

"What are you looking for in there, doc?" said I, wincing in pain.

"Always on the look-out for the odd rectal cancer," he said. "And, of course, in the mature male, one can expect an enlarged prostate. Mr. Podges, do you ever get lost?"

I told him I got lost after Violet died, and also when the New York Yankees swept the Oakland A's for the American League championship. He said he meant lost physically, like when I went for a walk did I find my way home all right. I told him I don't walk except to go some place I want to get to.

He wanted to know what my allergies were. "Alas," I said, "I have only the one allergy, and that is to the lowly Bermuda grass that thrives so well all over California."

How about daily physical exercise?

"Getting up and down from my chair," I said, "and thrice a week lightweight workouts on the famous Nautilus machines that are usually tackled only by athletic stars."

"Mr. Podges," he said, "I have the sense that you are on the whole quite indifferent to what's going on in the world outside you. Who is the president?"

"The president of what?" I inquired. He gave me a nasty look and wrote something down in my folder.

"I am not indifferent," I said, "to the fate of the Oakland A's, the 49ers football team, the Cal basketball team, and the Great Depression that is about to wipe us all out. I am not indifferent to doctor bills—*how much is this going to cost me, doc?*" You're not supposed to mention to medics anything vulgar like how much the bill is. The doc reared himself up to a dignified height. He put on his listening set and started tapping on my chest.

"I note," he declared, "that you are wearing one blue sock and one gray sock, Mr. Podges. How long have you had difficulty in locating your socks?" I told him I never wore socks or shoes around the house unless it was cold enough to freeze your balls off. And, I said, "when I go outdoors I like to experiment with what I wear—to have socks that match is no fun for anybody."

He asked me, "How do you sleep?"

I said usually on my right side but sometimes on my left side but sometimes on my back if I've just had a marvelous dream, but never flat on my stomach.

The doc said what he was trying to find out was how many hours a night I slept. I said I never counted them.

He asked me again did I have trouble finding my way home at night.

"Maybe I can't," I said. "I find myself frequently wandering into the Trauerkloss' house next door, as I am madly in love with their blonde, fifteen-year-old daughter."

Doctor: In love, eh? Can you remember when you had your last erection?

Me: Erection of what?

The doctor let out a long sigh and looked at me with sad eyes.

"Mr. Podges," he said, "what is the difference between a boy and a girl?"

"Not much difference any more," said I. "Girls nowadays wear dirty Levis they picked out of the Salvation Army's castoff clothes box and they cut their hair like Marines. Boys use deodorants and go to hairdressers to try to look pretty."

"That's all?"

"Isn't that enough?"

He made another note in my folder and asked me did I have my dizzy spells in the morning or in the evening. When did I last break a bone? How many of my ancestors died of cancer? Did I take any medicine for my headaches? Did I get upset when my heart missed a beat?

I answered every question with "Yes." The doc gave me a funny look.

"Look at my watch," he said. "What do you see?"

"It's a Citizen quartz chrystonic, made in Japan, costing you a fortune."

"No, no," he cried, "look in the little window, Mr. Podges. What do you see in the little window?"

I said I saw some numbers.

"And," he said, "what are the numbers that you see in the little window, Mr Podges?"

I said I saw 11:22:09 but, I said, "the truth is that time doesn't always go along with your watch. The only real clock is what I decide is a long time or a short time. Like this time here for your investigation is four to five hours long, in my clock."

He wrote something in his folder. The nurse called him out of the room so I peeked in the folder. I saw he had written "time disorientation."

When he got back in the room, I mentioned that I had to get up and pee two or three times a night.

"Yes, that's part of it," he said. I asked him what it was part of. He put his hands in his white pockets and swallowed a couple of times. "Part of the problem of growing older," he said. "The organs simply do wear out. Usually the kidneys go first and soon after the liver, and on to the lungs, the larynx and so forth. Piece by piece we are dismembered." A grim thought came into my head—I admit that. "And the pecker," I said. "Does that go, too, doc?"

He looked angry. "I thought you forgot what an erection is, Mr. Podges," he said.

"How could a fellow forget that," I declared. "So far my pecker is hale and hearty, although sometimes lazy. My question was, *does it go, too?*"

"Yes, the—uh—genitalia do slowly degenerate in the senior citizen."

"Fine by me," said I, "long as I don't lose my balls."

I forgot to tell him that I didn't really mind all that peeing, and that on a warm night I'm likely to go out in the backyard and piss under the stars, and I love the splash as much now as I did when I was a lad of six. (Marge caught me once when I risked a daytime pee behind the honeysuckle vine and later I heard Jack tell her, "it would seem that Hiram has entered the first stage of incontinence.")

I asked Doc Fimright if he studied psychology when he went to the school for medics. I had forgotten that doctors don't give patients the right to ask *them* questions. The doc smiled (sort of) and took out his pen. "I'm giving you some medicine," he announced.

I asked him what was the disease he had uncovered in me. "The prescription is for Dicumarol," he said. "It will help you adjust to your condition." I inquired as to what my condition was, which caused him to clear his throat and fold his arms. "Nothing to worry about, Mr. Podges—you're perfectly normal for your age. You may dress now. Would you like me to send the nurse in to help?"

"Oh do that!" I cried. "I can get *out* of my pants most easily, but it's real hard to get back into them without someone sympathetic to help. Please be kind enough to send in the red-haired one."

The doc gave me another dirty look.

While I was waiting for the elevator, I filed the prescription in the post office slot that's alongside the elevators.

I Discover the Vacuum

THE IDEA THAT I'm constantly about to drop dead is not confined to the medics. Take the case of tennis. I love to watch the tantrums of John McEnroe on the TV. I always had wanted to play tennis. Better late than never. I got a racket and yellow balls and signed up with the Oakland recreation folks for lessons.

When Jack got wind of this, he had an "at-your-age" talk with me. I wasn't to run fast on the court. In fact, I wasn't to run at all. If I couldn't get to the ball by walking, I should let the other fellow win the point. He said my heart might act up. I told him my heart was actually a muscle and a muscle doesn't like to lie around like a lazy cat. I told him the doc couldn't find any leaks in my heart. Jack declared that poor old Sandy Grieg dropped dead on a tennis court only a week after he had his electrocardiogram. "Listen," he said, holding his finger straight up as if he was the Pope, "if you ever get to the stage where you play somebody, never play more than one set. Don't forget, I am responsible for you."

Needless to say, I have carefully concealed from Jack the fact how I go to the club and lift the various Nautilus weights.

I am not supposed to do the things that they do between the ages of twenty and fifty.

Each passing year got me better settled in the full bloom of my creative senility. (Pablo said that's a "mixed metaphor," but how else could I say that? Pablo also said a famed psychiatrist once said, "Don't push the river—it flows by itself." That was already my idea, even before Pablo told me that. Unfortunately, the people outside of you think you're half dead if you just float with the river. But that's why this book is a story.)

You may remember how Aunt Jessie had this passion for bringing me flowers. Well, my chopping up the carnations was *not* the end of it. Oh no!

Only a couple of weeks later she spotted me in my room lost in the delights of *Sports Illustrated* magazine—and she cried, "Hiram, you must not shut yourself away like this. There are vast acres in the hills where you can take long walks that will improve your circulation and restore your vim and vigor."

"Thrice a week," I declared, "I go to the club and work out on the Nautilus machines. I also have a sauna bath and thereafter a gay time in the Jacuzzi tub. When I work out on the machines, there are hundreds of strong, pretty girls improving their figures nearby me. But please don't tell Jack because he worries about my heart."

"That is just a drop in the bucket," said Aunt Jessie. "You need to get into an overall mind-body complex. Long walks are what created the great British empire."

"And look at it now," I said.

She grabbed a chair and sat down on it very close up to me, and she took ahold of my hand. "Hiram," she said, whispering fiercely, "at this stage of your life the enemy is inertia."

"I walk," I said, "only when I have a place I want to get to. I walk to the BART station to get to the A's games. I walk to the bus to get to Cal's athletic contests. I walk in San Francisco so I can observe the rich people showing off their expensive clothes outside the palatial restaurants. When Teddy and I are outside, we do crawling races sometimes and I can beat him, although I usually let him win by an inch or two."

The only person Aunt Jessie listens to is herself. She folded her arms and said, "Hiram, it simply does not do your mental health any good for you to be alone so much." Only a few blocks from my house, she revealed, there was a senior citizen station where I could go to learn how to weave baskets or make lovely pottery and meet fascinating folks my own age.

"I already know too many people," I said. "I do not have a yen to make pottery. We already have too many dishes in the house. And I am willing to leave basket weaving to the Indians, who doubtless need the money from selling them to rich tourists."

"Very well," she declared, "then you can learn to paint. Paint in oil! Big, expressive canvases! No, that would cost too much. Then paint in watercolors, Hiram. Bring back the old days in Iowa. Pay tribute to that wonderful era when Violet was alive and life was so full for you."

"Every time I open my eyes I paint a picture," I said, "much better than anything a paint brush can ever do."

"You could give them as Christmas presents, dear. It will take you out of yourself. It will!"

She was dancing up and down with her dyed red hair jiggling with enthusiasm for my artistic future.

"I hardly ever think much about Iowa," I said, "and why should I want to be taken out of myself after all the time and trouble I took to get into myself?"

"Flowers, then!" she cried. "I know how much you love them. You can paint them all. Chrysanthemums! Delicate yellow roses! Lilies of the valley!" She took my hands and pulled me to my feet, and I felt a tremendous yen to get my point of view across to her.

"One thing I have noticed," I said, "is that flowers do not give a darn whether or not you paint them. What they like best is when the bees have intercourse with them."

"Intercourse?" She heard *that* word.

"Yeah," I said. "Flowers and bees like sex as much as we do." She is the wife of a Presbyterian elder. When I saw how pale her face got, I felt sorry that I had to do that to her.

Feeling sorry for her is really not necessary—she bounces back from whatever catastrophe hits her. She stayed for dinner that night and it so happened that a spoonful of peas didn't quite make it into my mouth and a couple of peas rolled merrily down over my shirt buttons. Eagle-eyed, she tugs at Marge's sleeve and points at my wandering peas. Aunt Jessie has some mysterious power over Marge, who obediently cried "Hiram!" and pointed at the peas as if they were dog-do. If you're over the age of sixty, they score all the mishaps in your life and tote them up as further proof that you're about to shuffle off their mortal coil.

The other night Marge made us some cold soup made of white fungus, sour cream, soy bean sprouts and Chinese herbs, from a recipe she got at a workshop on *Zen and the Art of Tummy Maintenance*. Jack dearly loves Marge and therefore managed to keep sipping. I just had to spit my mouthful back into the bowl. "Hiram, don't be childish!" cried Marge. Meanwhile, Teddy had poured his milk into his soup and was about to dump what was in the sugar bowl into his bowl when Marge caught him. She gave him a forgiving smile.

"I'm childish, too," Teddy said, and grinned at me. He understands.

Let me point out that one dark and chilly January day—Teddy was about age three then—he was looking out of the window at the dreary rainfall and he turns around and grins at me and says, "There's sunshine in my soul today." At that moment I *knew* what I'd already

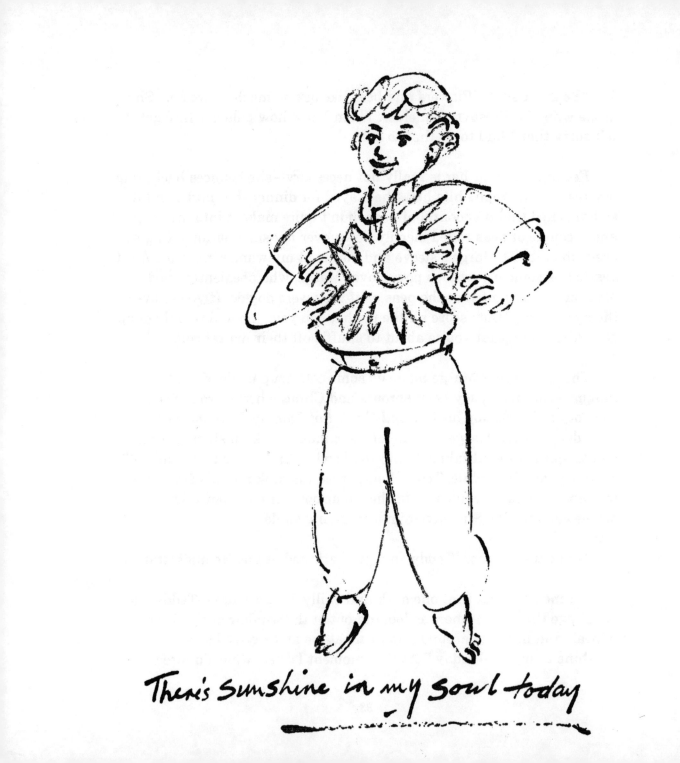

There's sunshine in my soul today

suspected, that Teddy and I had some kind of a secret telegraph system going between us. True, both of us are second-class citizens—but there's more to it than that. Let me try to explain better.

One day I was all alone in my room. You know how it is that, when you close your eyes, there's always something you see or something you hear or you touch or you smell. I had just started to turn on my TV when I got a yen not to do anything whatsoever at all. I got to wonder what would it be like for me to be dead. I started thinking about the yogi I read about once in *Life* magazine, some guy from India that they wired up to fancy instruments and told him to stop his heart from beating for five minutes. He was famous for doing that. They wanted to find the secret of how he did it, but they never did. I wondered, was he a dead man for five minutes?

I was thinking about this fellow while I was sitting there and I closed my eyes and it got very black. I mean black-blackety-black—nothing to see whatsoever, and I didn't hear a single thing. It seemed like I had gone away somewhere without my permission. Maybe it was like ending up in some incredibly big vacuum.

Alas, it only lasted for a second or two. It's hard to use words about. It's maybe like lying on a white cloud and floating way up high and out into the blueness that gets black as it goes way out past Saturn and Jupiter and all that. And there's not a cloud left to lie on. I even forgot there was a me to lie on it. But I was there.

Even though it was a vacuum, it wasn't. There were all these galaxies and I was the supreme commander of them, and at the same time I was a little tiny thing like a poppy seed, so little and wrinkled up you'd never believe it had life in it anxious to grow up and be a poppy in the sunshine.

When I started coming back out of the vacuum, I felt even happier than I used to just after lovemaking with Violet, and better satisfied than if I had eaten all the hot fudge sundaes ever made. I was setting the rules of what I am, not the other way round.

Who is going to believe me when I say, which is the truth, that in this situation I was more me than I was when I was twenty, thirty, forty, fifty, sixty or seventy years of age? You don't have to stay long in the vacuum because there isn't any time in it. I know that sounds goofy and it even sounds goofy to me right at this moment. I have been darned careful not to tell a soul about this, not even Marge. Well, I did mention it to Pablo. He said there was proof in literature that others have this experience—for instance, Mr. William Wordsworth, the English poet. That made it respectable for me. Well, there was another time that I got into that vacuum when Teddy, who was age four by then, came into my room. When I opened my eyes and looked at him, the little fellow jumped into my lap and looked straight at me and hugged my arm while smiling.

He knew!

But who wants to stay in a vacuum? The other day I went to the Oakland flower show. The fuchsia display had a net around it to keep the hummingbirds in, I guess. While the birds dived in and out of the magenta blossoms, I burst into tears. A young lady rushed over and put her arm around me—"What's the matter, dear?"

"I just find it most wondrous," I cried, "that these superstar birds actually exist and that these flowers love to be strafed and I am allowed to be here seeing the whole thing, paying only $1.50 admission. Honey, don't take your arm away."

I blush to confess this to all of you who read this book, but what else can I do, since creative senility is exactly what makes such a thing happen.

Once Again, the Third Degree

IT HAPPENED THAT ONLY A few hours after that vacuum business between Teddy and me, Jack came home from the City in one of his study-Hiram moods.

The longer he studies geriatrics at the Med. school, the more I get to be his favorite guinea pig. Right after dinner he calls me into his room and takes out his notebook. He wants me to tell him what is the capital of Ohio (which, as every schoolboy knows, is Toledo). I replied that obviously the capital was Cincinnati or Cleveland. "Um-hm," says Jack, or words to that effect. He smiled at his notebook and asked me how did I know that. I replied, "Cincinnati has the Reds and Cleveland has the Indians, which both are highly regarded ball clubs, except this year. You couldn't make a town like Akron the capital. Could you?"

"Now listen to me very carefully, Hiram," says Jack. "I want you to try to think of the name of the device they used for weighing food when you were in the prime of your life."

"Scales," I said.

"Yes, Hiram," he said, "and who made the scales?"

Me: I seem to recollect that in Iowa City the scales of Mrs. Wilson's store were bought from a fellow named Fritz Bruncke or was it Fluncke.

Jack: Hiram, old boy, what was the name of the company—you know, what corporation was it that did the manufacturing and put its name on each and every scale in those days?

Me: Toledo.

Jack: Great, Hiram! Wonderful! Now is there any connection, any connection at all, between the name of that company and the capital of Ohio?

The way he asked the question made me feel dumb. I just shrugged my shoulders and he scribbled in his notebook.

Next he wanted me to tell him what was the population of New York City. I said I'd only been there once and that was probably in June of 1951, and Violet was along. No, it must have been on our twenty-fifth wedding anniversary, which would make it around 1958.

"So," said Jack, "what was the population of New York City when you and Violet visited it?" I replied that from what I saw of the place the population would come out at a hundred million.

"Too many folks there," I explained, "who needs to count them? They're piled up high in the sky and stacked like miserable sardines in underground cars—they have to cut each other's throats to get some breathing space. Oh! I've got it—Toledo is the capital of Ohio." I thought that would overjoy him, but he frowned at his notebook and scratched something out.

"Here's an easy one for you, Hiram," Jack said. "Tell me what does the Census Bureau do?"

I scratched my head. "It's an outfit in Washington," I said.

Jack: Right!

Me: I reckon its job is to try to bring us back to our senses. Jack closed his eyes and let out a very sad sigh.

Next item: What month are we in now? "What matters," I said, "is if it's summer or winter. What matters is whether leaves are falling or there's snow that has to be shovelled so you can get in the door or whether it's so hot you have to close all the blinds and hole up with cold lemonade in order to survive."

He scribbled in his notebook.

Whoever thought up the system of twelve months, anyway? I just had to tell my true thoughts to Jack. I told him, "The names of things probably don't matter as much as you think they do. Didn't Shakespeare say, 'What's in a name?'" Jack smiled at me the way he does at Teddy. I was lovable, but I wasn't supposed to be taken seriously.

"Who is the president now?" Jack asked.

Oh no, not again!

"The president of what?" I asked. He said, "The president of the United States, of course, Hiram." His idea is that if you're born in a certain country the president has to be the president of that country. So if you were born in the U.S.A., the president of France doesn't matter a hoot, or even the president of General Motors.

I just had to speak this out. "Jack," I declared, "it does not matter to me who the U.S. president is because what's the difference between the Republicans and the Democrats. They both make a mess of everything. What does matter is that we're hell-bent for another Great Depression and the price of whiskey has tripled, denying great joy to the common man."

Jack made quite a long note in his notebook and then he said, "Hiram, please just answer the question. Now *what was* the question, please?" "Didn't you ask me who caused the price of whiskey to triple?" He shut his notebook. I asked him what grade I got. "It's not like school," he said. So I asked him what was the point of the test. He put a fond arm around my shoulder. "Hiram, old boy," he said, "don't feel that you're a failure. You did just fine. Just fine."

But his face looked really sad. I knew he had lost some money playing the stocks, and that he'd just invested in a new company called Computersports and he had high hopes of making a killing. I felt obliged to cheer him out of the sadness I had caused him.

"Jack," I said, "I sure hope that Computersports turns out to be a good friend to you."

I really did hope that, because when he looks sad he looks just like the ten-year-old kid I knew in Minnesota when I was just his Uncle Hiram and he felt bad because his mother was very sick in the hospital.

The Glad Hand Attack

As YOU CAN SEE, creative senility is not considered to be your birthright. An example of this was the TV show, "Over Easy." It was designed for old folks. Their idea was that you have to "cope" with senility. They tried to teach you how to keep the undertaker from the door. Never will you catch them calling anybody old. Maybe they think old age is a disease, except in the case of French wines, Italian violins and Scotch castles.

I recollected the days when you had to whisper the words "syphilis" and "gonorrhea." The papers called them "social diseases." The word "homosexual" was a state secret, but nowadays in San Francisco the word "gay" is celebrated proudly with civic parades and with half-naked photographs all over page one.

Furthermore, it's bad taste to die of cancer. The newspaper obituary columns say "after a long illness."

One night while I was watching the A's on TV, I heard this top-sergeant's voice yelling at me from the living room. *Aunt Jessie!*

93

She gets more vigorous every time I see her. She has gone and gotten a new wig that makes her hair sort of blonde, and she has it short the way boys' hair used to be, and also the way the Berkeley lesbians wear their hair.

Jessie walked over to my TV and turned it off. "You don't need that, Hiram," she declared. "TV is what they use in convalescent homes where the elderly are put out of sight." She declared that she read in *The Chronicle* a study about persons who make it to be a hundred years of age. She said they discovered that these people all had reached outside of themselves, stayed active in the community and did things constantly with bodies and minds. "Hiram, dear," she said, "the fact is you are drifting dangerously toward becoming a shut-in. We don't want that now, do we, Hiram?" She took ahold of my hands and pulled me to my feet and steered me into the dining room. She had a lot of printed stuff laid out on the table.

"I have given a lot of thought to you lately," she declared. "Sit down. What I have here for you is the schedules of events for the senior citizens as devised by Vista College. I've circled in red the courses that will be helpful to you in your situation."

She put her thumb down on a red circle. "This course is mandatory," she said—*Movement With Ease for Older Adults.*

I explained to her that three mornings a week I go over to the athletic club and use their Nautilus machines and their Jacuzzi fountain. "Lots of movement," I said.

"*Movement with Ease* begins at 3:30 p.m.," she said, "the very time that you so often daydream on the back porch. And look at this one, dear—*Writing, Remembering and Dreaming* at the Albany Senior Center. They will give you homework that will help you cut down on the mind wandering."

I am at last getting the idea that the best thing to do with Aunt Jessie is to let her get the wind out of her sails because in her enthusiasm she always—well, usually—forgets all about what it was that she started out to reform you to.

"Here's the one that's my very favorite for you, Hiram," she cried, "*Serendipity and Chutzpah in Confronting Life-Threatening Illness.* That's the mystical side of your situation, and chutzpah is the Jewish way of being brave and we must admit, mustn't we, that the Jews have been very brave."

I asked her what did she mean by my "situation."

"Oh," she said, "the usual concerns about getting cancer, kidney failure, about how much the arteries have hardened, about the wrinkles and sagging flesh, the sleepless nights, the forgetfulness, the varicose veins, the feeling of being left out."

I told her I hardly ever had the time to give those topics a thought.

"Of course you do, dear!" she cried, standing on tiptoe and slapping me on the back. "No need, no need whatever, to hide your fears from me, Hiram." She put her finger on another red circle on the Vista College schedule. "*Song Writing Workshop For Seniors.* Wouldn't it be grand," she said, "for you to write some songs about how your life turned out?"

"It hasn't stopped turning out," I said.

She seized my hand in both of hers and said, "You could sing out your memories of the old Iowa years, the school days, athletic feats, the courtships, the. . . ."

"Jessie," I said, trying in vain to pull my hand out of her grip, "if I ever wrote songs I'd write them about the folks that tell me 'you don't look a day over fifty' and the folks that mess up my hair and say, 'Stay in there, sport, you're good for at least ten more years,' and the ones that try to help me get out of automobiles. A song about. . . ."

"Hiram," she said, and squeezed my hand even harder. "These negative thoughts pile up because you get cut off. At this stage of life, dear, the enemy is inertia. In that study of people over a hundred years old they found. . . ."

"I already read the whole thing," I said. I finally got my hand out of her grip and grabbed my stomach with both hands.

"Excuse me," I cried, and ran to the bathroom and locked myself in. After a couple of minutes she was banging on the door and asking if she should send for the doctor.

"I love it in here," I said. "I'm going to have a hot tub bath and languish in it. I am going to use up all of Marge's lavender bubble soap. Maybe I'll write a song about a hundred-year-old weight lifter who got elected president of the U.S.A."

When I came out of the bathroom, I saw that Aunt Jessie was over on the Trauerkloss' back porch, sitting alongside old Fred. It looked like she had the Vista College schedule in her lap and was showing stuff to Fred.

She blew me a kiss and put her arm around Fred. I sure did wish her all possible luck in getting him to sign up for the class in *Serendipity and Chutzpah in Confronting Life-Threatening Illness.*

The Shrink and I

CALIFORNIA IS ABOUT AS different from Iowa as a baby wren is different from a pelican. I sure learned that during my first five years out here. For one thing, everybody in California simply has got to have at least one expert all his own. I overhear these gals yakking with Marge. One talks about "my acupuncturist." Another one talks about "my bioenergeticist." You hear it at parties, too. Even some of the men. There's "my Shiatsu masseuse," "my astrologist," "my Gestalt therapist," "my yoga teacher," etc., etc. One of the favorite experts the women have is "my psychic." A psychic is the California word for what we used to call the Gypsy fortune tellers that came through Iowa. The other day when Marge's friend, Eloise, and another gal came calling, I just had to speak to them of "my palm reader." Their faces went deadly pale with shock. Says Eloise with her face outraged, "There are no palm readers any more, my dear. There are, however, tarot card readers." Marge smiled sweetly.

"There has been much progress," Eloise explained, "since you were a lad."

I must say, though, that Jack is not a hundred percent Californian. He sticks to the old-fashioned notion that science can handle every possible problem. Just last week he rushed into my room to announce that I had been chosen to take part in a "very significant project." I sometimes do wonder just what they mean by "significant." Maybe it depends on what your job is. For example, the U.S. Secretary of Defense argues that huge piles of atomic guns and missiles are significant. The bigger the pile, the more significance. I, with no job, don't find *anything* to be specially significant. I admit that I like, or even love, the walnut squares and almond royals produced by the See's candy stores, but I wouldn't dare call them significant. Even the way Teddy and I get along now that he's age six, I wouldn't call significant—it is just Teddy and me getting along, nothing more and nothing less.

Maybe calling something significant is a way for a fellow to say he thinks that he's more important than the next fellow.

Anyway, I asked Jack, politely, "What is this significant project?"

Jack: It's a project that will be a milestone in geriatric history.

Me: I hope nobody will try to stick his finger up my butt.

Jack: Not to worry, Hiram, he's not a medical doctor. It's a project headed by Dr. Klaus Bonesplat, an eminent research psychologist. And I will be there to hold your hand, old boy.

Me: That's nice.

Jack: You will become a pioneer. Fortunately for you, Dr. Bonesplat is short on senior citizens for this project.

I concluded that this was a golden opportunity for me to compare my own researches with those of the famous experts.

Dr. Bonesplat had his office over in Frisco in one of those new-fangled buildings you see in fancy-Dan neighborhoods these days—hundreds of glass walls and potted palms under spotlights and statues of naked people trying to look noble. The waiting room was full of charts on the wall showing Dr. Bonesplat's various diplomas.

He wears designer spectacles, and he is very tall. He showed me into his office like I was a guest of honor at a White House affair. He grabbed my hand and held onto it and said he was delighted that I was going to work with him. I said I remembered seeing him on the "Over Easy" show on Channel 9.

"Ah, yes," he said, "I do what I can to try to smooth the path for the elderly." He steered me into one of those expensive leather chairs where your ass sinks down six feet. I must say, that *did* feel significant.

"Now," he declared, "I'll hold up a big card. Look at it and tell me what you see. Don't think—give the first answer that comes to you."

He held up a card. He had spattered black ink all over it—making a mess like when your fountain pen leaks. What I saw on his card was a baseball stadium full of Yankee rooters in the golden era of Joe DiMaggio. When I told him what I saw, he said for me to try again. I figured he wasn't a Yankee fan, so I tried the National League. "It's the

Giants versus the Pirates," I said. "The Giants are ahead two to zero, top of the ninth, and as is usual with the Giants, the Pirates now have got three runs in the bottom of the ninth and have won the game 3-2. All those little dots are Giants fans going wild with shame."

"Aha!" Dr. Bonesplat folded his arms and stared at me as if he was the school principal.

He asked me did I have high blood pressure and I asked him how did I do on his test. "Mr. Podges," he said, "*no*body has ever before seen a crowd of people on this card." He looked at me as if I had taken a crap on his pure-white linoleum floor. "You see a crowd," he said, "because you feel lonely and cut off." I said I never felt any such way except after Lillian left on Thursday nights after I've given her help with her school studies.

Jack came over and laid a hand on my shoulder. My shoulder gets a lot of laying-on of hands in this era of my life. "Hiram," says Jack, "it will work out better if you just are honest with Dr. Bonesplat."

"Take your time," said Dr. Bonesplat, "and don't hestitate to share your innermost feelings, Mr. Podges."

"All right!" I cried. "I love to sit in the sunshine all by myself with no boss to tell me to do this or to stop doing that. Glorious freedom! I revel in the sports events constantly on TV and who needs company for that. I revel in all the secrets that Teddy and I have together. I also revel in Marge taking me sometimes to help her shop in the supermarket. Drama! The kids fighting their moms for a piece of candy. . . ."

"Hold it," he said, and put his spectacles on the end of his nose and stared down at me.

"You said I should share from the heart," I said. "Let me say, Dr. Bonesplat, that it is important for your researches for you to know that the older I get the less I like to be in a crowd getting pushed and kicked around, except at the A's games and Cal basketball and in Frisco watching the Gay Lib parades and the ladies parading around Berkeley for equal rights and the 49ers celebrating their football triumphs. . . ."

"That will *do*, Mr. Podges," he declared. "All I need is the gut responses to the cards."

Jack comes over and lays a kindly hand on my shoulder. "Hiram," says he, "don't feel that you have to hide your inner fears from us."

The psychologist said we would try another card. This time the black blobs were even wilder and unfortunately what I saw was New York City going up in flames—millions of people melting because unfriendly planes had dropped a couple of H-bombs on Times Square, which is at the center of the city.

When I told that to Dr. B, he got a chair and sat down opposite me. "Mr. Podges," he said, "it is quite understandable that, at your age, you should have fears of everything coming to an end." He faced toward

102

Jack and said, "This is an instance of the projection of geriatric fear that is clinically very significant."

"Doc," I said, "I'm not afraid to die, if that's what you're driving at."

People just don't like to hear you say something like that. Dr. B's Adam's apple kept going up and down with nervousness. "Of course you're not," he said, "of course not."

"Doc," I said, "you know why I saw that terrible scene on your card? It was because purely and simply that is what's going to happen to you and Jack and your kids and Marge and Teddy, as well as me and the dog, if you youngsters don't stop playing chicken with the Russians."

This time the sympathetic hand on my shoulder was laid on me by him. "Mr. Podges," said he, in a very silky voice, "all of us have fears as we go through life. When we can't face the fear inside, we do what is known in science as 'project' it onto some person or some object outside. These cards were designed to catch your projections. A projection is seeing outside the ugliness that has been dammed up inside. In your case you have projected your personal fears onto the national defense programs of President Reagan and his Secretary of Defense. Let me hasten to assure, Mr. Podges, that is *quite* understandable—you are perfectly normal for a person in the sunset years.

A brilliant idea came into my head.

"Doc," said I, "I have a brilliant idea for teamwork between us. How'd you like for me and you to do this on one of those TV how-to-cope shows. You'll show a card to the TV millions and I'll cope with it and then you'll explain how I'm projecting all my fears of death, pain, grief and the other standard disasters. We'll show them that the things they cope with at home, such as rheumatism or the gout or athlete's foot, are nothing when compared to the hidden horrors these cards can unearth in the senior citizen. This will cheer them up wonderfully. Thus your research project will become a great social benefit and. . . ."

Jack rushes over to my easy chair and pulls me onto my feet.

"Hiram," he says, "I'm sorry we have upset you."

Dr. B looked very hurt. He took my hand, and at the same time that he kept saying "thank you, thank you," he was ushering me out through the doorway.

My Very Best Friend

SO I FLUNKED Doc B's tests. I went over to Berkeley that afternoon and had a beer with Pablo. I confessed to him that I felt sorry I had not let Jack make much "geriatric history."

"Not to worry," Pablo said. "*They* are the ones who flunked. They are the ones who think old age is a disease."

Pablo, more than any grown-up I know, is someone I believe. He is a profound thinker, just like the famed statue by Rodin, the French sculptor. For example, Pablo told me once that if the United States was a person he would be locked up in the booby hatch as too dangerous to be left loose.

Speaking of flunking tests, I recall that as a kid I thought flunking was a disaster. "Nothing succeeds like success," "the impossible is possible"—those are the Iowa mottoes I was brought up on. There was a jury inside me—I called it "they." Whenever I had an impulse to do something, "they" decided whether I should or shouldn't. Lucky for me I caught on even before I was thirty that "they" didn't really know what I wanted.

To tell the truth, flunking can be as much fun as passing. One of the grandest gifts of senility is not to have to pay attention any more at all to what "they" think the score is. ("They" keep score.) In fact, you're surrounded from birth by people who want you to do what "they" want.

In my case there *is* one person who understands about this and that person is Teddy.

One Christmas morning when Teddy was four, Marge and Jack and assorted relatives and hangers-on all sent expensive toys to Teddy, and on Christmas morning Aunt Jessie and Uncle Charlie, her husband, and their kids and others assembled to watch Teddy do the unwrapping. He started to unwrap something when he saw an orange lying under the tree. Boy, he went for that orange as if it was the Taj Mahal! That's all that he wanted, to play with that orange! This made the yuletide audience furious. Didn't the little fellow know the meaning of Christmas?

Guess they'd have to teach him—Jack grabs a present, the biggest one, and sets it in front of Teddy, saying in a sweet voice, "Teddy, see this string? If you pull the string, the wrapping will come undone and you'll find something very wonderful inside—and all for you!"

Teddy was surrounded by smiling adults who could hardly wait for Teddy to do it. What he did was give his dad his angel smile and keep right on making love to the orange. The kid was cut off from reality—premature senility at age four.

Then Marge moves in to try with her sweetest mama role. No progress. As you know by now, Aunt Jessie loves a situation where her unconquerable spirit is the only hope. She realized that Christmas morning would be ruined for all present (except Teddy and me) if Teddy kept on doing what he wanted to do.

"Teddy, Santa has sent me to be your helper," she cried, and guided his tiny hands into pulling the strings, as required. When he sat among all the exposed gifts, he went back to his orange and you could see that for him the orange was the whole universe. Even today, now that he's six, he still doesn't have that "they" jury inside him, as far as I can tell.

I'm probably the only one that sympathizes with Teddy's senility—his "poor attention span," "occasional incontinence," forgetfulness, over-emotionalness, etc. His senility is forgiven by the grown-ups because he'll "grow out of it." But me—I should "know better after all these years."

It's obvious he and I were meant for one another. Lots of days he doesn't go out to play, just so he can hang around me. He's almost independent of what "they" want him to be. Like they think he has to go to the zoo, but when I took him there he couldn't stand seeing all the animals in jail. He cried so hard I had to hug him hard to calm him down, and then rush him away from all the cages.

Teddy doesn't have the faintest idea of how much he knows. Or maybe the truth is he doesn't know much about knowing, so he just lets everything be whatever it happens to be.

The other day he came in towing his plaster alligator, Hercules, that has wheels under it.

Me: Teddy, you never brought Hercules to visit me before, did you?

Teddy: I was scared you wouldn't like him.

Me: Scared—of me?

Teddy: Hercules is *bad*.

Me: You like him a lot, don't you?

Teddy: Yes, yes, yes.

Me: I think it's OK to have a friend who's bad.

Teddy: Do you have bad friends, too?

Me: Uh-huh.

Which probably was a lie. One difference between Teddy's senility and mine is that he's hardly yet begun to divide things up into good and bad. When he says "bad" he usually means "good," too. I had to live for seven decades before I found out it was a waste of time to always decide one thing is good and another thing is bad. Pablo's not even thirty and he's got the idea already. What he says is "we are all one." It's hard for me to concentrate on that idealistic idea when I think of Lew Sodhunter. Why would I want to become one with a guy who does a hundred push-ups every morning and thinks if you don't do the same you're a bad citizen?

Teddy *likes* Lew Sodhunter. Which shows you he is ahead of me.

Teddy has got very dark red hair. His eyes are as blue as Lake Tahoe is, or should I say nicer than turquoise. He's got dimples. Just to look at him makes me laugh. He's got a secret he can't tell you. Sometimes he grins and looks sort of sideways as if he saw some huge, all-powerful angel grinning back at him.

We don't use words but we communicate secrets, like I said, on a secret telegraph system.

I told Pablo that although it embarrassed me to tell it, the truth was I thought *Teddy* was an angel—a real, live angel right here with us on the earth. At least most of the time.

During the ensuing conversation, Pablo asked me why did angels fly. I said because they had wings. "Also," he said, "because they take things lightly."

I think that covers the situation between me and Teddy—even when he's bad, he's good. I remember the time when he figured out how to get to the top shelf in the kitchen and raided Marge out of her last jar of the wonderful gooseberry jam that Aunt Jessie's husband made, and it was Jack's favorite. Jack and Marge had a long huddle about whether

Teddy had stolen the jam. "The question is," Jack said, "has he developed sufficient ethical sense yet to know he must not take other people's property."

They decided he had not been bad. If they had voted for him being bad, they would have punished him.

The truth is, Teddy did not actually finish off the jam all by himself. He brought it into my room and said, "I found a nice present for us." I rushed into the kitchen and got the crackers and we had a feast.

I'm in Love, I'm in Love, I'm in Love

YOU MAY RECALL THAT earlier on I claimed that forgetfulness was the finest flower of them all. Well, it is a fact that as more time goes by *everything* does change. It took me more than four years in Oakland before I got to fully discover that the really finest flower of them all was second childhood. It's even better than first childhood! Yes! *Because you can combine your young childhood with your second adolescence!* That is to say, I can play blissfully with Teddy some days, while on other days I can have my joys of watching the young beauty queens cavort on the Cal campus. And sometimes I can do both on the same day. What an embarrassment of riches!

I was seventy-two years of age, or was it seventy-three, or was it seventy-four, when the seeds of my second childhood gathered themselves into one beautiful spot and shot up out of the earth in the form of my intense interest in Lillian, Fred Trauerkloss' winsome granddaughter. She was fifteen at the time, and so were my feelings toward her. When I was age fifteen in Iowa, I had a terrible crush on Ella Mae Roosevelt (no relation to FDR). That was terrible because I was so shy I couldn't get up the nerve to speak to her, and if she cast a glance my way I got so hot and bothered I had to look the other way. Terrible as that was, it was, I confess, wondrously mysterious—and it covered the whole world in a carpet of the brightest of colors and it made all food and even the air I breathed taste like dessert, and it made me sigh like that poor lovesick lad I saw on the TV in *Ah, Wilderness!* The truth is, such sighs are terrible pains that are made of noble longings no poet could put into the human language.

So that's the way I was with Lillian. *But without the pain!* I knew she usually came back from high school at about 3 p.m. and I tried to be on the front porch every day to watch her glide past me on her bike with her blonde tresses shaking golden showers upon the sidewalk behind her. Let me assure you this was far better than it had been with Ella Mae by reason of the fact that it wasn't painful. That is to say, with Ella Mae my heart fluttered with a million plans for our lovemaking—some of these plans, I do admit, had her naked in the bushes with me and we did as many of the naughty things as I could think up. So it was painful to want all that and to be nowhere near getting it.

But with Lillian, considering that I could be her granddad, my body lust did not consume me, simply because it could not be part of the picture. So my joys of watching her were not painful! Just pure old-fashioned joy!

I was out there on the porch most every school-day afternoon, shy and happy. Through the autumn and the spring and also on the chilly winter days. For months I said nary a word to Lillian. I guess she took me for just the old man next door whiling away his last hours in memories of a life gone by. I guess a whole year went by and then I heard from Fred that Lillian was now in the Far West High School, and she came home a little later —about 3:30 p.m. She would ride her bicycle past with her books and her makeup in a canvas bag on her back. I watched and as she pedaled nearer and nearer the joy in me of my heart beat faster and faster every day.

I spoke no word to her ever. I could have been the mailbox. But one afternoon she threw a hello my way. I felt great, great gratitude.

Young love! It's the best kind—you feel it and she doesn't have to feel it back for you, although it sure is easier if she does.

Lillian tossing me that hello made me into a can of gasoline with a lighted match thrown into it.

This went on for weeks. Fortunately, for all concerned, each week the fire in me got quieter. I guess Lillian must have decided I was just a harmless, if friendly, old fellow and nothing to run away from because finally it got so that she'd stop and talk to me almost every day.

Lillian *shone*. I mean her sweater, if it was red, was redder than red usually is. And her tennis shoe, one foot on the step as she balanced on her bike—that foot shone like a Bible halo.

All this commotion inside me and the shiningness outside fortunately did not keep me from listening to what she said. I really listened. She told me she adored the study of economics. She said the

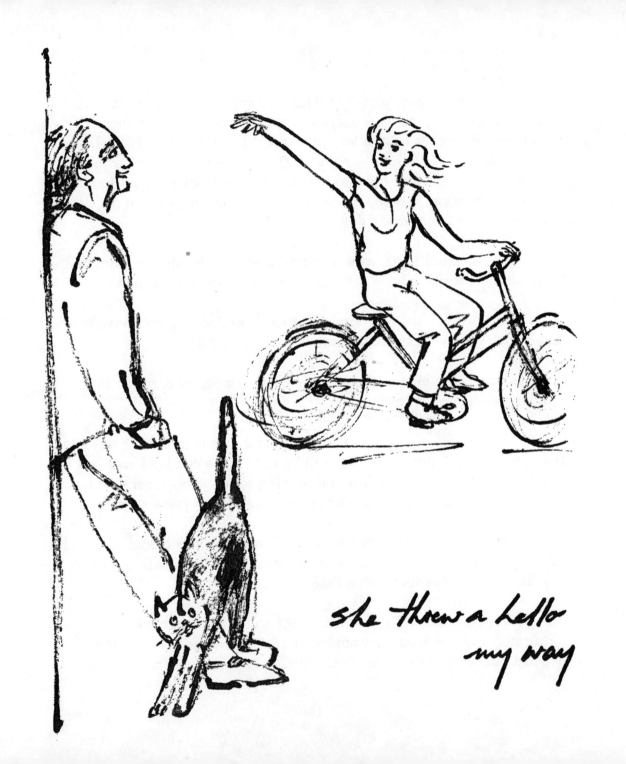

she threw a hello
my way

depression that our country was in for demanded that people learn about economics so they could forecast better and make all the budgets match up. She said she felt great sorrow that her father did not believe girls can make good economists. I told her boys and girls were equal except on tennis courts, football fields and the muscle-building machines.

It got so she considered me pretty much a confidant. For instance, she told me her boyfriend, Al, the basketball star, was always trying to get her into bed with him whereas she wanted the sex part to wait until they got really well acquainted. She said the girls at Far West High School thought she was a Puritan, and asked what did I think. I said, "Follow your heart." There is the advantage of being senile—if you use the word "heart" to a young girl you won't be scorned at for doing so. To tell you the truth, Lillian liked my saying that. She said she once read a book she loved that told about a Mexican witch doctor called Don Juan who advised, "follow the path that has heart." She thought it was "incredible" that I should use those very same words. In any case, she started telling me even more secrets, which it would be unfair to disclose to the public. Finally, she confessed to me that the study of geometry was almost unbearably hard for her. So it ended up with her coming over every Thursday night for help with it, and I am proud to say I kept my mind on isoceles triangles and such, even while my heart was acting up like the Calaveras jumping frog.

It got so she stayed on for an extra half-hour sometimes.

Second Adolescence

LET ME SAY RIGHT HERE that if you're over the age of sixty and adolescent, people treat you the way they treat alcoholics. You're laughed at for things you'd otherwise get killed for, such as when I poured my champagne over Jack's head last Christmas and he gave me a dirty look but instantly forgave me because of my senility—which was actually just an act of plain old second adolescence.

When you have your first adolescence, the grown-ups think all your sighing and moaning and not being able to eat and your living on the moon day and night— they think all that is something to be gotten over with. Bad enough for a kid, they think, but surely for an old person unthinkable, absolutely out of the question.

So there was I, innocently floating high above the firmament in the full bloom of my second adolescence when the cruel outside world cast its dark shadow over it all. *They* think I should have gotten over young love sixty years ago. You know how parents laugh at a fifteen-year-old boy when he's in love—it can't be deep unless an adult feels it.

116

I am sorry to report that Marge, bless her soul, was a party to this kind of attitude. There were some times when she was not my friend.

She sat me down for her version of the at-your-age talk. "Hiram," says Marge, "some of the girls (that is, the coffee-klatchers) have noticed that you have developed, uh, a certain, uh, enthusiasm shall we say in connection with Lillian Trauerkloss.

"Oh yes!" I cried. "Yes, yes! It's true! It's true!"

Marge has a pretty face and I hated to see her lips compressed and all tight the way they were. She was hurting. I wanted to tell her I was in love with Lillian but I didn't dare to. I wanted to say, "Marge, you don't have to screw somebody to love her," but I didn't dare.

What I said aloud was, "My interest in Lillian is, alas, from a great distance. Sometimes after the Thursday night sessions she puts her arm around me and kisses me on the cheek and thanks me for knowing so much about geometry. I, however, have never touched her."

Marge: Hiram, that's under*stood*. What concerns me is what's *appropriate*.

Me: I recall that Mr. Charlie Chaplin, the famous movie comedian, flourished from the companionship of very young ladies.

Marge: Good heavens, Hiram, I hope you're not having thoughts like that.

Me: I don't *need* to touch her. Just being two feet away from her makes my heart beat faster and my body is fifteen years old and I smell the lilac smell from the yard in Iowa City and I hear my mom and dad fighting and I am in my room safe from all adults and I am the supreme creator of the universe and I am chewing gum. Actually, the *Reader's Digest* says moderate exercise is good for the heart. When my heart beats for Lillian, it gets stronger.

I realized after it was too late that I had let out such a wondrous display of words that Marge might think I was daft. Indeed, she promptly left my room. She couldn't cope with the eloquence of my senility. Nevertheless, I felt a little bit ashamed just the way I used to when I was a kid and my masturbation got spoiled by the hygiene talk by the gym teacher who said that when we woke up in the morning we should rush off and take a cold shower so as to kill off any impure thoughts.

But I never could stay ashamed for more than a minute.

Marge hadn't been to church for years, but I forgot that a born Presbyterian can't completely stop being a Presbyterian. After that talk Marge saw to it that Lillian and I sat in the dining room for our lesson, in plain sight of all.

It was a game we were playing, just as much as checkers is a game. Marge's last move was to be very cool to Lillian, never ever offered her hot chocolate, as though to discourage her from coming over.

When the Cat's Away,
the Mice Will Play

THE OTHER BIG GLORY OF second childhood comes out for me via Teddy. As I mentioned, part of our friendship comes from our both being second-class citizens.

I remember how mad Marge got at Teddy once because he had figured out that by standing on a chair he could reach the peanut butter and he ate half of it. When she told Jack about it, he told Teddy to "march right up" to his room and go without his supper. He suffers when he's treated like a slave. Jack and Marge don't ever confine me in my room but they hardly ever treat me fully as an equal.

My friendship with Teddy has gotten to be a delicious and natural flow like the way real Vermont maple syrup is when poured onto melting butter that's on piping-hot buckwheat cakes.

I don't know just when what was best between us began to be. Maybe it was when Teddy was about age four. He began to play with himself one day and Marge rushed over and pulled his hand away from his private parts and slapped his hand and he cried.

Jack and Marge used me quite a bit as the baby-sitter and one afternoon when Teddy and I were upstairs in his room he started up again playing with himself. He looked over at me. He was waiting to see if I would come over and stop him. I was thinking of what I heard one of the Iowa lit. professors say—that Mark Twain had proclaimed that "morality is what feels good." Golly, that little guy was feeling *good*. I looked the other way—if I grinned at him he might tell Marge. Next time I looked he was still doing it. I remembered how much fun I had as a kid playing with myself. I found out about it one day while trying to learn to ride a bike. Later on I got to looking for playmates to do it better with.

Teddy kept looking at me and it just hit me that he would never tattle on me to Marge, so I winked at him.

A big payoff from being senile is you can't remember to be ashamed whenever something feels good. I confess right here that I still play with myself every now and then, and I have gotten pretty good at it. Deep down somewhere, I bet, Teddy knew that why I winked at him was to tell him I did it, too, though I don't imagine he guessed that I thought of Violet when I did.

So Teddy and I had the same secret feel-good practice. There is nothing better to promote friendship than to have a secret with somebody that you can't even tell to your own mother.

Marge caught Teddy doing it again and of course she had to go tell Jack. Pretty soon they had Teddy's hands in weird sort of gloves "so as to break the habit." The next time I got to be the baby-sitter I took the gloves off him until Marge and Jack got to the front door.

We do various secret things. The other night when they went bowling I was drinking some B and B. Teddy begged for a taste. I mixed some of it in ice cream and gave it to him. He wanted another one. Of course it's not supposed to be moral to give alcohol to little kids but I figured this was just a B and B sundae. But, as it turned out, Teddy was a little bit tipsy when they got home from the bowling alley. "My," Marge said to him, "you *do* look bright-eyed." Teddy said I had told him a very nice story (which was not a lie).

Jack and Marge gazed at me with gratitude.

That was about the time that Teddy had his period of playing doctor and nurse with LaVerne, despite the fact that when Marge caught them at it she scolded Teddy very hard and tattled to LaVerne's mother about it. LaVerne lives just across the street. She is just about Teddy's age. LaVerne's mother is a Jehovah's Witness and, boy, did she carry on about her darling daughter being subjected to such a game.

When Teddy is the doctor of course he has to remove some or all of the patient's garments in order to check for diseases. When LaVerne is the nurse of course she has to check for diseases so as to have something to tell the doctor about.

Sometimes when Teddy is sure LaVerne's mother is out of the neighborhood, and Marge is out of the house, he'll go get LaVerne and start up the game. I take up a lookout station on the front steps and if I detect danger I call back to the kids, "Alle, Alle hanson free," so they can make themselves respectable.

I don't care if you think I am being bad, being the guard. The truth is that all creatures, large and small, like to know all they can about how other creatures are made, and males and females have a lot more to be curious about each other. You can learn a lot more about it playing doctor-and-nurse than by sneaking looks in anatomy books.

I guess Teddy must have been about five when we played lots of games just for the two of us. Sometimes when I went for a walk he would come along with his red wagon. I sit in the wagon and he pulls me. The other day he pulled me all the way over to Guy's Drug Store. One lordly gentleman stopped us and frowned at me as if I was a criminal.

"What is the matter with you?" he asked.

Me: Nothing, thank you.

Gent: If you're not sick, why should this little tot have to pull you?

Me: I pay him one Tootsie Roll for each ride.

Gent: Did you know that's against the child labor law?

Me: Tootsie Mootsie.

Teddy offered to give the gentleman a free ride. The gentleman strode off in a huff. I'm sorry to say that most adults are like that.

Playing can be fun even when Teddy's not along. Like I was with Marge once in Capwell's dignified department store, while she was purchasing a nightgown, and I went over to the bra department and told the salesgirl, "I'd like to look at something that will make my wife look sexier." She glared at me for daring to use such a word at my age. "I assume," she says, "that your wife is somewhat younger than you are." I pointed proudly at Marge, who's about half a century my junior. The saleslady blanched with the shame of my robbing the cradle.

If an old man is too outrageous, all he gets is curses, and sometimes they even sentence him to one of those convalescent homes. A kid who is outrageous always gets forgiven in the long run.

We are very lucky in our house that our Teddy is an angel most all of the time. But he has his outrageous moments, and they are creative. If you tell him he has to eat his mashed carrots, he's highly insulted and will do art work with them on the plastic table cloth. Marge's lectures about the starving people in Bangladesh do not interest him in the least. Yesterday he picked up a dish of spinach souffle' and hurled it to the floor. Thereafter he waited for the slap on the wrist, which is a small price to pay for all the self-expression. While being slapped, he lets out a loud wail and studies Marge's face. He wails until he sees she's feeling she was cruel—and rushes over to hug him.

People have awfully romantic ideas about their own first childhoods. When I listen in on some of Marge's coffee klatches, I hear the wildest tributes being made to their childhoods. Marge can't get enough of telling how marvelous the homemade peach ice cream was at her eighth birthday party—"It was real, thick, organic farm cream, something you never find any more in the store." And Ellie raves about how wonderful the colors were in those days, *so* exquisite, *so* bright and all the smells *so* sweet. My, my.

"Oh!" cries Marge, "I shall never, ever forget the magic of that languid summer morning when they gave me my pony, truly a sensitive, bespeckled animal friend. My very own!" (Marge reads novels.)

They go on and on about the joys under the big Barnum and Bailey Circus tent, the glorious thrills of playing blindman's bluff at dusk, the magical mystery of bedtime stories read by mommy or Uncle Do-Dad, the delicious taffy pulls and, my, your taffy was *simply coal black* from the dirt you forgot to wash off your hands.

Never, ever again will it be that way!

But when you get into second childhood, don't expect any medals. For instance, I have always all my life liked to skip sometimes on the sidewalk. There's something about skipping that beats running or walking. But if I'm out with Marge and start skipping, she pretends she's not with me.

On a hot day I'll buy at least one black-walnut-banana ice cream cone. The fellow hands me the cone with a look that says, "At your age!" I also like to wear bright-red sweaters, but people think bright red is a color only for people under age thirty-five.

The other night we had beet greens with vinegar at dinner. They were trying it out because Lew Sodhunter informed them it was *the* way to build up vital minerals in the body. (The people of California are always busy building up this or that in their bodies the same way they're always looking for gurus to lead them to Oriental salvation.)

As soon as I bit into those greens my gut felt under attack. I just spit it back out into the bowl. "What's the *matter?*" cries Marge. "It's not poison," says Jack. He forgot he's studying my senility. Neither of them bothered to notice that Teddy had used his beet greens to decorate his bib even before I spit mine out.

I Cultivate Mind Wandering

I HEARD JACK TELL Marge that mind wandering is the "first clinical evidence of senility." "Clinical" is how the medics say you have actually caught a mind in the act of wandering.

The opposite of wandering is being stuck in one place. So if your mind gets stuck in one place, you're normal, and if your mind takes off like a space rocket, you're out of the human race. One afternoon on the Cal campus I heard this fellow in Hindu headgear speech making. He said a thought travels 166,000 times faster than light does. Well, we all know that light is full of wanderlust. So thoughts must be even more so.

Teddy has now become a six-year-old. Being with him shows me it is natural for the mind to wander. For instance, I was telling him about how Alice got into Wonderland by having the gumption to go into a hole in the ground. Teddy jumped up and down, clapping his hands, and he rushed into the backyard. But he couldn't find a hole there and he came back to my room weeping. I concentrated hard on some way to find him a hole. Meanwhile he was yelling at me to open my mouth wide. I did so. And he says "wider." And he jams his head against my mouth and cries "hole, hole!" And he's laughing. He had let go of the whole big Alice In Wonderland deal because in this new game we didn't even need to leave the room to find a hole.

If he had been a grown-up, he would have stuck to his passion to find a hole in the ground. And since there was no hole in our backyard he would have been miserable and sad all day long.

Mind wandering allows you to let go of some loads of stale and worn-out ideas and let in something new and fresh. When Teddy gets into a regular school, they will train his mind to stick to one subject even when it hates the subject. They did that to me—that's why I never bothered to finish high school. You have to ditch the training you got in school.

When I'm on the back porch, sometimes I get on the magic carpet and take off. I've seen the Grand Canyon at sunrise and the famous Taj Mahal in moonlight. I've had a beer with Winnie Churchill, the British war leader, and I've played golf with Sinatra and beat him and I also beat the U.S. ex-presidents who constantly go to Palm Springs. I've been in bed with Marilyn Monroe and Jean Harlow. I won the bobsled tournament in the Olympics. I got lost in a Sahara sandstorm and was rescued by a team of brave French schoolgirls who nursed me back to health. I started to run for U.S. president once, but on thinking it over I gave up the idea because who wants to be shot dead?

In the days when I was working in Iowa City I could hardly let my mind wander at all. Too busy. And when I got home at night Violet kept bringing up topics of such burning interest to me that my mind got stuck on her topics.

I only started getting good at mind wandering a few years after I moved in with Jack and Marge.

I realize that Jack doesn't like to have me talk too much during meals, and I understand his viewpoint. Husbands and wives like to have the center of the stage when the husband is away all day. I try not to butt in too much. But this time I couldn't hold back making remarks about Jack's "clinical evidence" of senility. I told him just to really look honestly at his own mind. I told him that if he went in the bathroom and sat down and looked at his mind he'd see what a jitterbug it was. (The bathroom is the only room in the house where privacy is a sure thing.)

"Jack," I cried, "just close your eyes in there and *watch* and you'll see your mind acting like a Mexican jumping bean. Jack, you don't think that stuff up, it comes all by itself. It's your mind and it wanders and so does everybody else's mind wander all the time. Minds love to wander. That's where those great ideas came from Jack. Think of Thomas Edison, think of Marie what's her name, the queen that lost her head."

"Marie Antoinette."

"Think of Christopher Columbus. Think of Woody Allen. Think of. . . ."

"Enough!" Jack cried. He looked vexed, and being vexed upset him because he does his darnedest to be the scientist toward me. He pulled himself together enough so as to give me the same kind of smile he gives Teddy sometimes, like he did yesterday when Teddy parked his fire wagon in the kitchen, and when Jack said to "get that thing outside," Teddy said the kitchen was now the garage for the fire wagon and it was the wagon's bedtime.

This type of Jack smile says he understands the very old, and the very young, have a right to their irrational behavior as long as it doesn't mess with the adults' life-style.

He laid his hand fondly on my shoulder. "Hiram," he declared, "you have to understand that you can no longer expect to keep pace with the world around you which, at this stage of your life, seems to be moving too fast for you to participate in it. Your mind wandering is a wholesome retreat for you—it serves to make you feel more powerful and less helpless. Please understand that we don't criticize you for this in any way, Hiram. But don't kid yourself into believing it's natural for us, too. How do you think I could get through medical school if I ever let my mind wander?"

Part of him was especially vexed with me for suggesting that he use the bathroom for his mind wandering.

"I *know* how my mind works," said he, "and I *never* sit on a toilet seat except when I have to."

129

I was glad I spoke up, for thereby I got a lot of attention from Jack and also, I hope, planted a seed by which he might learn to every now and then let the universe carry him with it, and by which he might not have to wait, as I did, until the age of seventy-three to start his mind wandering.

It's Fun to Weep

WHEN PEOPLE CELEBRATE THEIR birthdays, what they celebrate is getting through another year without total disaster. I used to want to skip my birthdays but Violet always wanted to whoop it up, so what could I do? Marge always goes in for that, too, so when June 29 rolls around, there's the celebration for me. This year was the biggie—age seventy-seven. There was more than the usual gifts of stuff you couldn't possibly need, or that you already have, and the one golden candle signifying seventy-seven. I blow out the candle on the cake and they cheer like I'd scored a touchdown and sing the happy birthday song which is not much of a tune but Teddy loves it so I do, too.

Jack decided to get very chummy with me, which is a rare treat. He asked a lot about his mom as a kid and did his dad really believe in the Bible and how many boyfriends did his mom have before her marriage. Meanwhile, Marge is coming and going with all my favorite foods and stroking my head and cooing and kow-towing. She told me, "You're really just a big adorable overgrown panda." If you're a panda, you don't have to be taken too seriously. Jack even got into asking about my dad and Daisy, my mother. I tried to answer all his questions even though those folks don't mean any more to me nowadays than does Woodrow Wilson and other such people who have gone out of existence just as much as people you have in your dreams.

Lillian came over to be our baby-sitter, and Jack and Marge took me to the movie of my choice, which was an old one called "Julia." There are some scenes in this movie where Jane Fonda and Vanessa Redgrave are in a lot of trouble together in Nazi Germany and I just couldn't keep back the tears. Jack grips my shoulder hard as if to say I should get ahold of myself. Men just are not supposed to weep *and certainly not in public*, although it is true that great he-man football players weep and shamelessly slap each others' fannies after their Superbowl victories. But that comes under the heading of patriotic deliriousness so nobody complains.

As a rule, though, *old* men are allowed to weep, in their senile weakness, just like little kids are. I guess that in the theater Jack forgot to study me and therefore he got embarrassed by my shameless public deportment.

To tell the truth, I cry a lot more than I used to, partly because I have more time to get emotional in than when I had the faculty club job. Anyway, Violet did enough weeping for the two of us. It made me nervous, but to tell the truth she enjoyed it.

My dad had a rule that boys must not cry. I broke the rule secretly at sad movies, making loud coughing noises to deceive nearby girls. I admit I cried pretty hard watching Jack Kennedy get buried on TV and didn't care who noticed. I cried even when I saw Sadat, the ancient enemy from Egypt, walk down the red carpet in the Holy Land—I thought Egypt and Israel were going to kiss and make up. Senile idealism!

When I was a kid I cried when dad gave me a surprise ticket to the Iowa-Minnesota game. But I waited until dad was out of sight.

I don't say that I cultivate weeping, but if some sad memory grabs me when somebody is around, I don't mind the attention I get. If Marge is around she'll come over and put her arm around me and say something like, "Oh, Hiram, dear, what *is* it?"

The other day I recalled the tragic occasion when I was six and my Airedale, Bowser the Third, got run over in front of our house in Cedar Rapids.

The truth is that it's fun to weep when you're sad. Think of how everybody enjoys getting sad at the movies—the worse the catastrophe the better.

In the case of remembering Bowser, a couple of tears fell out and Marge rushed to my side. I did not tell what made me cry—Bowser was not a friend of hers. Anyway, when she came back from shopping she brought me a chocolate eclair with real cream in it flavored with real rum. She knows it's in my top-ten list.

Except for desserts, I have less of an appetite in my "golden years," since I no longer have to do things like play handball constantly to prove I'm a man. Marge keeps piling stuff onto my plate and I keep shoving it back. Even Jack looks nervous when I refuse to eat like a horse.

My being skinny constantly worries Marge. "You're so *thin*," she told me, and looked at me as if *rigor mortis* was about to set it.

"So was Gandhi, the great Indian diplomat," I said.

I also told her that at my age it's normal to have "a failing appetite." The word "failing" gets to her and so she requests me to name some delicacy that might arouse my digestive glands. Recently I have been treated to blueberry cheesecake, walnut croissants, not to mention Beck's imported beer with soft pretzels. On my pension pay I can't afford stuff like that. Neither can Jack and Marge.

Will Wonders Never Cease!

THERE'S ONE THING I have found to be an eternal and undeniable truth—
that the human being is capable of giving you any kind of surprise.
*Any*body can change. Take the case of Lillian's grandfather, Fred
Trauerkloss. As I explained, he had turned himself into what he most of
all feared he'd become, a parsnip. He was the last person in the world
that I'd ever think could get a chance at creative senility. So imagine
my surprise when I saw him on the street *two blocks away* from his
house. He was walking arm and arm with Aunt Jessie. Not only that,
they were traveling fast while chattering to one another. I could not
help but cry out, "Fred, where are you going?"

He stopped walking and smiled at me. *Smiled!*

Fred: I am going to my Wednesday class.

Me: What is it you're studying?

Fred: The main subject is "chutzpah." That's the Jewish word for
bravery. Once you learn it, everything else changes. You tackle new

tasks, such as archery, which is now my favorite hobby. On Sunday Jessie and I are going sailing on the bay, along with her son, Randy. Come springtime I shall plant me a huge veggie garden that will be free of deadly preservatives and lethal chemicals. All this comes from the study of chutzpah.

Me: How do they teach that to you, Fred?

Fred: They use serendipity, mainly.

Me: Sarah who?

Fred: Serendipity is not a lady, Hiram. Serendipity is figuring a way around the hardening of your emotional arteries. I'm sorry, Hiram, we'll have to run along or we'll be late. I don't want to miss a minute of it.

Me: Jessie, are you in this class, too?

Jessie: I just go along for the sheer joy of watching Fred blossom even as do Japanese paper flowers when one puts them in water.

Fred: Ta-ta, Hiram. See you in church.

Me: So long.

Fred: Don't take any wooden nickels.

All I can say is, one man's meat is another man's poison.

It took me over a week to get over the shock of Fred's big changeover. Then I began to ponder on just what it was about Aunt Jessie that made me back away from her when poor old half-dead Fred experienced a miracle by *not* backing away.

I asked myself, was I drifting away, like Lew Sodhunter said I was? Was I letting myself get too private?

I saw a television show on the life of Dr. Carl Jung, the famous psychologist. It seems that he thought half of us are introverts and the other half are extraverts. He argued that an extravert looks for what's important in the outside world and has to have other people around to make him feel he's somebody, and he's always doing something, such as giving a party. This psychologist said the introvert thinks that what goes on in his head is the best part and he loves to be alone a lot and he can just be.

This got me thinking about old Fred and me. All his life he was a super extravert—he was president of his class at the Far West High School, he was first-string quarterback on their football team, he was the debating champion, and when as a lad he got his first erection, he could not wait to try it out in some girl and thereafter, even after his marriage, he flitted from dame to dame like some drunk horsefly.

So it was goldarned awful for him when his body began to get old and he could no more be the champion in athletics and sex.

Thinking about this, I just had to decide that I surely was and still remain a confirmed introvert. I love people just as much as Fred ever did—but *one at a time.*

I was congratulating myself on how superior I was when I glimpsed Fred in his backyard planting his rows of sweet corn for the summer's crop. His cheeks looked rosy and he was whistling "I've been working on the railroad, all the live-long day."

Well, I just *couldn't* feel superior to him. I decided, what the heck, I'll just give him a shot of extraversion.

"Hi, Fred," I cried. "Looks like you're going to have some dandy corn roasts this year."

"Yessir!" cried Fred. "And you're invited, Hi."

I always thought the name Hiram was nickname-proof. But here, for the first time in my whole life I heard myself called by a nickname. I was Hi Podges, Jr.!

"Come over and have a beer," Fred shouted.

As we imbibed together he told me all about his plans for growing tomatoes, lettuce, zucchini squash, string beans, etc.

"I took a cooking class," he said. "I specialize in the Chinese stir fry, using a wok of course, and pure vegetable oil. As you probably know, meat is lethal."

I asked him what was all the lumber stacked up against the back porch. "I'm going to build me a redwood hot tub," he said, "and you're invited to come sit naked with us."

I got to thinking about Aunt Jessie's vigorousness when, it seems like, Fred read my mind.

"All of this new life-style I owe to Marge's Aunt Jessie and the Vista College crowd," he cried. "She is a *doll*."

You Just Never Know. . . .

THAT CONVERSATION WITH FRED took place a couple of days after my seventy-fifth birthday party—and only a few days before another event that was a real big shock for me, to put it mildly.

The March of Time radio show used to say about people, "as it must to all men, death came yesterday to—" Sure, we all know that we'll all die, but when I got the news on the phone I thought it was a specially mean practical joke. The news came from Aunt Jessie's husband, Charlie. I answered the phone. He said she was felled by a massive heart attack and died.

"Oh come on," I told Charlie, "there must be some mistake—she's never had a sick heart." I argued with him as if he was too dumb to get things straight.

When I looked in the *Tribune* there it was in cold type—"beloved wife of," "beloved mother of," fifty-six years of age. I went down and walked around Lake Merritt, around and around trying to get it to be a real fact.

I guess the truth is that Jessie was the type of person you can't think of as dead. They had her laid out in a coffin, the way Presbyterians do, down in some cold-blooded funeral home, but I couldn't get the heart to go look at her for I knew how undertakers try to make a dead woman's face look like a star in a burlesque show.

Golly, it sure is funny how I had forgotten the many cozy hours she and I spent together. They sure do come back to me now, though.

A year before she died—hell, I can hardly write down that word about her. It was a year before that that she and I had a walk in the rose garden in the Berkeley hills—a place she was crazy about. She told me I was the only person she could trust to keep a certain super secret. Her secret was that her husband, Charlie, had been having a love affair with a lady of the church choir, and it had gone on for years. She said she never told Charlie she knew.

"I even wore different-colored wigs to try to get him interested again," she said. "I've tried to make up for it by giving extra love to everyone in the world."

That was the only time I saw tears on her face.

I put my arm around her. And I did cry, just a little bit. She pushed my arm away. "I don't feel your arm is sincere," she said. "But I thank you for the tears you shed. No man can manufacture tears that are phony. Some women can, but no man can, ever, Hiram."

She had done her darnedest to try to make me into her ideal senior citizen. She cared. She cared too hard so I backed away and she went next door and put her ideals onto Fred. And it seems like maybe he's carrying her energy now—he's found a lady friend in the Vista College senior citizen sculpture class.

Jessie told me once she believed Fred was in love with her but kept it secret because she was married and a good Presbyterian. It's a fact that love doesn't always obey the law.

The last time I saw Jessie I was sitting on the back porch observing a squirrel. She winked at me and said to Marge, "Hiram is the immovable object and I am the irresistible force." Maybe that meant she thought I had a perfect right to be an introvert.

That got me to thinking about Violet, who sure was an extravert. I always took her for granted. As though all her good looks and her famous rhubarb pies and the special smiles for me had been just what I was entitled to.

She had lots of pain in her last months, but as I told you she died with that real special look in her eyes as if she'd just come outdoors for the first time and saw what sunshine looked like.

I also got to thinking about what Pablo said, that angels fly because they take things lightly. Can you imagine an angel flying around with a heavy knapsack on its back? Or carrying a steamer trunk? Or even an attache' case?

I first got the idea of having less stuff when I left Iowa City. I gave away huge piles of crap. I got it down to two suitcases full, and *that* was too much. In Chicago I leapt aboard the train to Oakland and, boy, was I flying lightly. More is not better, except when you are starving to death.

Even More Than Neighborly

LET ME TELL YOU one more delicious item.

It started on a sun-drenched Sunday morning last May. I was out back under the elm tree admiring the buds when Marge rushed out of the house and confided to me that she and Jack wanted to have a private breakfast and could I take charge of Teddy.

Surely man and his mate require a heart-to-heart talk now and then.

They proceeded to have their eggs Benedict and chocolate croissants on the back porch while Teddy and I tried to find his rubber snake. He dotes on the snake and if he thinks it got lost he goes crazy. It's a snake locked up in a cardboard box that leaps out in anger when you unhook the lid of the box.

I did not especially try to snoop on Jack and Marge but I confess I heard her tell him, "Sometimes I think Hiram knows certain things we don't know." It so happens that this idea of hers came out of a conversation she and I had a while back.

As I no doubt have mentioned to you, I often like to sit on the back porch. Just sitting.

When I'm on the back porch all alone I don't have to keep looking at my watch, worrying about some place I should go to. I enjoy how neighborly everything is. One day while sitting I was watching the Trauerkloss' black cat with her muscles all coiled in her jungle game of hoping she could grab the robin that was playing innocently on the moss by the pond. The sunshine felt good on my face and it suddenly dawned on me that the same sunshine was heating up the robin and the moss and the cat, too. That's what I meant by it all being neighborly. Well, let me confess—even more than neighborly. I *was* the robin, too! And I was the cat and the moss and the sunshine heat! Don't tell me I was just imagining—I *knew* I was all that as well as my own self sitting in the wicker chair. Meanwhile, the cat caught the robin and feathers flew. I was the hurt the robin felt and I was the cat's great joy. Good grief, I was that, too!

I had to tell somebody about it because I wondered if I was going crazy. I phoned Pablo but he was down in Los Angeles giving a lecture, his girlfriend said. I figured Marge was the only grown-up around who might not laugh at me for confessing this. So I just plain told her about it. She has very big and very comely hazel-colored eyes and when she's in a good mood they fill up with honey. She just listened to me and let it be what I said it was and her eyes filled up with honey. So I just outright told her also about the time when I was sixteen and broke my

145

leg trying the high jump, just to show the girls I was as good as Jim Blakey. Well, I landed with one leg crunched under me and it broke and the pain got terrific, and I just went up in the air about ten feet and watched them run for the doctor. Up in the air away from the pain I didn't feel my leg hurting one bit, so I stayed up in the air where it didn't hurt. I could see my body writhing in pain but I didn't feel it and I could see their sympathy and I tried to yell at them, "Hey, it's OK, I'm up here, it doesn't hurt a bit." The doctor came and gave a pain shot to the me that was down there on the track field.

I decided it was now safe to come back down into my body, and so I did.

When I thought about it later I just had to ask myself who was the I that was up in the air and who was the I that stayed on the playground. Did I live in my body or did my body live in me? Ah, sweet mystery of life!

Meanwhile, Teddy found his beloved snake under the living room davenport. Inasmuch as Teddy was fascinated by his snake friend, I just let myself be immoral—I just shamelessly tiptoed to the kitchen so I could hear more of what they were saying on the back porch.

I overheard Marge tell Jack, of all people, all this stuff I've just told you about. What a catastrophe! I guess she hoped Jack's medical science would explain it all.

"Nothing to worry about, dear," says Jack, as I listened in from my room. "These notions are typical of the confusion endemic at that age."

(Later I looked that word up. The dictionary gave an example—"typhus is endemic in certain countries.")

"At the age of sixteen, too?" Marge said. "He wasn't senile then, was he?"

"In adolescence," Jack declared, "hormonal changes and emotional confusion about identity produce such phenomena. In second childhood the adolescent delusions tend to erupt again, as in the case of Hiram's identity getting mixed up with that of the robin and that of the cat."

I peeked at them from behind the frig. I saw Marge put down her croissant and stare at it.

"The fact is," said Jack, "that after you're thirty your brain loses 100,000 cells every single day. On your thirtieth birthday *you'll* start going downhill." He was looking off into the sky, making calculations in the clouds. "So far," he announced, "Hiram has lost on the order of 500,000,000 brain cells."

"Good heavens!" cried Marge.

Then I heard Marge say, "Jack, I wonder if *my* brain already has a leak in it." Her voice was trembly and I feared she might break out in tears.

I peeked again. He had his arm around her and was tenderly kissing her. "You're only twenty-seven," he said, "and you're very, very beautiful and in your right mind."

"Jack," she cried, "I just have to tell you that sometimes when I watch Teddy play with the doggie I get almost the same exact feeling Hiram said he got with the robin and the cat."

I was thinking that sure was something to make him flip his lid—his own wife getting senile. But no—he just told her calmly, "Not to worry, honey. It's simply that the motherhood instinct took you back to the period when you were pregnant and you and Teddy indeed were pretty much one."

"The puppy," she said. "I wasn't pregnant with the puppy, Jack."

She is so polite to him.

"Well," he says, laughing, "maternal protection overextended to *Canis Minor*." It turns out that's a fancy expression he must have picked up in medical school. The dictionary says it means "little dog."

There was a long silence—and suddenly Marge is telling him she remembered that when she was a girl she went for walks in the woods and that one time in the woods she had a distinct impression that the trees and the squirrels, the jack-in-the-pulpits, and even persons and even her own body—and everything!—were just one single being. "Jack," she cried piteously, "I was only eight years old. That was before my hormones began to get shuffled around, and surely there were no big brain cell leaks, Jack."

That kept Jack silent for a minute. Then he says, "The ability to discriminate between inner and outer events develops with

148

acculturation. Look at how many delusions Teddy has. They're *cute* sometimes, I agree. I have no doubt that he experiences his plastic alligator as part of his own little ego."

"If Teddy's delusions are cute," she said, "why aren't Hiram's cute, too?" That was a very, very bold thing for Marge to say to her scientific husband. He did not answer the question!

Well, isn't that something—*Jack not able to explain it.*

Home Safe in the Empire of the Dolphins

THE HISTORY OF THE HUMAN RACE tells me that I, too, will die pretty soon. So I really appreciate the days and nights that come along. Each sunset is more interesting than the last one was because each sunset may be the last one. Little daily things get to be more important. So-called big things fade away. I used to get all wrapped up in things like should Roosevelt or Willkie be the U.S. president. I mean to say that my senility has shown me for instance that every moment in life is like a banana split that's given free of charge, and it's the only banana split left in the world.

Back in Iowa I always thought I had to do something all the time. That's what the schoolteachers tried to drill into me. I played a lot of blackjack with Violet, had endless debates with Olaf Svennson, trying to show myself smarter than he was, went bowling twice a week, went to movies constantly. Nowadays I have time instead. I like to sit on the back porch a lot. Time is my really very best friend. On the back porch I don't have to even believe there is a clock. Time stretches really far nowadays.

I secretly suspect that the human soul does not go anywhere when you die. Maybe the soul does not have to catch a train for a better place—maybe it just stays wherever it was when you started out. I thought about this when I saw the big tragic carrying-on about Aunt Jessie by Marge and assorted relatives and hangers-on. They wouldn't let go of her.

When I was twenty, even when I was fifty, I acted as if I was going to live forever in this body. OK. But I missed a lot by getting snookered a lot into planning and expecting. I say the future really doesn't exist until it starts happening. I remember there was a play once called, *You Can't Take It With You.*

Teddy does not bother to hang onto anything except a couple of very favorite toys. He doesn't hang on to yesterday, either—you don't hear him sitting around reminiscing about the wonderful birthday party he went to yesterday.

Jack and Marge are already bored with that life-size panda doll that sits on their bed daytimes (made in Taiwan exclusively for the Neiman-Marcus store). But I bet they won't let go of it till it begins to rot, or they do.

One day in January when Teddy was between age three and age four he was standing by the window looking out into a black, cold, rainy day, and he said, "There's sunshine in my soul today." Teddy didn't say it to me. He said it to the outdoors. But as soon as I rushed over to him, his big blue eyes looked at me and I felt sure he saw the sunshine in *my* soul.

Two or three years have gone by since that, and all I can say is that Teddy and I found lots of ways of proving in action how much we were together in soulhood.

One day when Teddy and Marge were out and I had the house all to myself, I turned on the hi-fi and put on a record called the "Bolero." It hit me that this music was made with the idea that whoever listened to it should not just sit still. I shed all my clothes and danced. With the Bolero you're led to go from slow-slow to insane fast-fast. You whirl and get very dizzy and every problem that ever existed anywhere gets shucked off in the whirls. Great success! I thanked the Bolero and then I put on the Poet and Peasant Overture. High drama! I danced all sorts of roles. I was the proud king bestowing favors on his humble admirers. I was a slave overjoyed with bowing low. I was a sensitive poet hiding from the husky peasant. I was a wild Iroquois warrior scalping the white invaders in Iowa.

The next time Teddy and I were alone in the house it occurred to me to invite him to have a dance with me. He joyfully assented. It turned out that it was even better when two do it. I never would have thought of letting someone dance insanely on my back the way he did.

I was amazed that when I bowed low in worship of him as the king, he loved being worshipped and at the same time I could tell he knew I was only kidding.

Or was I only kidding?

We did this lots of times. We got so we would sing sometimes—any sounds would do. We made up sort of a language just for our own little

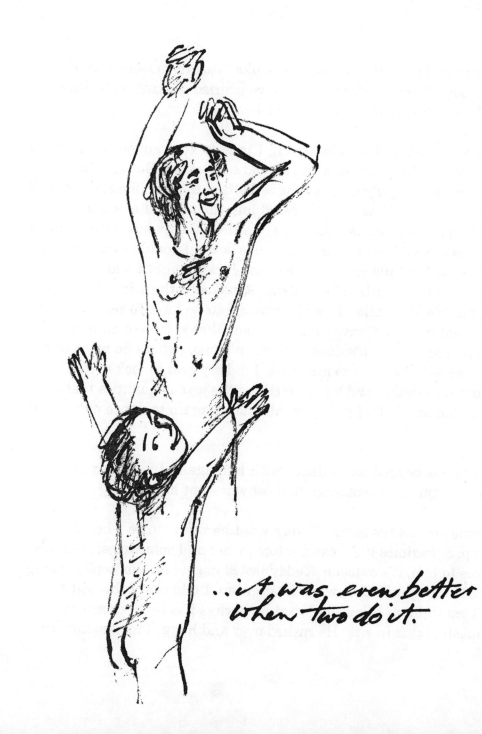

...it was even better when two do it.

tribe—sort of Hawaiian sounds, words like "stokansameensa" and "poopagushya" came out. Sometimes we whirled so hard we just had to fall down exhausted and laughing our heads off.

Since we both had our clothes off, I tried to keep an eye on the front door, lest some Presbyterian scout should be peeking. But one day Marge came home early and caught us both in the act. She sent us both to our rooms and told us to get dressed immediately. After Teddy was in bed that night, of course she had to go tattle to Jack about it. She made it sound as if we'd tried to burn the house down. I couldn't catch every word they said but the gist of it was that Jack thought I was supposed to be a "responsible citizen" and dancing naked with their kid was not a bit responsible. Jack told Marge he would hate to have to send me to a convalescent home. ("Convalescent" means that you have an incurable disease and are at death's door. It is not a home, either.) So when Jack came to me with his man-to-man talk, I did my best to look extremely sober and responsible and try to weed out the joyous qualities that are so disturbing to adults. I promised him never again to dance naked with Teddy.

Teddy has begged me to dance with him again. I won't give in. I sure don't want to be sentenced to a convalescent home.

People are always asking Teddy what he wants to be when he grows up. Sometimes it's a candy-store owner and sometimes, if Jack's been nice to him, it's a doctor. Teddy tested me out on this topic, asking me what I thought he'd be when he grew up. I told him I thought he would keep right on being just what he always has been, except for being much bigger in size. He rushed over and hugged me around my legs. Maybe he already suspected all that schooling will knock it out of him, his being exactly himself.

He asks me lots of questions. He asked me, "Did I come from out of my mother?" I said he did, and he asked, "How did I get into my mother?" Marge overheard this and rushed over to tell Teddy she would explain it all when he got a little older. The next time he and I were alone and he asked me the same question I said he got into his mother because he decided she would be the best person to be born from. He looked at me puzzled-like—and I grinned at him. Suddenly he's strutting around the room like Napoleon, saying "*I* decided where to start."

It has gotten to be that every word we say to each other is loaded up with all the secrets, and let me tell you our words are delicious. Even more delicious are the times when we do things without words. Like the time I was reading him something about dolphins, how amazing it is the way they coordinate their swim teams, and all that. "I am a dolphin," he said. It wasn't the words, it was the way his big blue eyes looked at me, giving me the idea that he had been or maybe even still was more than just a human being.

Thinking about his dolphin look I decided to carry on like a perfect grampa and lecture him on the importance of those first six years of his life, how he should keep the dolphin alive and kicking right up to the end. I went on and on. I admit I enjoyed feeling like I knew how his future should turn out for him. Teddy went out of the room and came back with his crayons and paper and started to draw. He drew the rear end of a human being so it looked like the fellow had gotten his head stuck in a hole in the ground. When I asked him what the picture was, he said, "It's the king. He's got a head too big so it has got captured by the gopher hole."

So much for my big head.

If Marge punishes him, he likes to go get his bubble set and blow lots of bubbles. He used to do it always alone, but one day he came into my room with his bubble set. A great honor! I asked him what a bubble was. He said, "It's what you want everything to be, and I never had a bubble that didn't get busted almost right away." He offered to let me blow some. I was blowing one when I heard a loud female cry at the front door saying "Yoo-hoo" and then, "Ready or not, here I come!" It was Aunt Jessie. (This was before she died.)

She said how delightful it was for us to be blowing bubbles. She sang us a line from "I'm forever blowing bubbles." She took out her pen and started poking into Teddy's bubbles. "See how nicely they explode!" she cried. Teddy ran over and jumped into my lap and sucked his thumb.

"You know, Hiram," she said, "bubbles are lovely. But do you realize this house hasn't a single educational toy?" She said she was going to buy Teddy a nice game he and I could play together that would at the same time be a lesson in "'primitive arithmetic." Teddy told her he and I already had plenty of games and they weren't lessons.

If Marge is out at night I get to be the storyteller. I made up a story about a little kid who wanted to be a hero—and in his own way, not the way the grown-ups thought he should. This boy went on an adventure into a strange land far from home where he met an old man who was the king of hearts. The king protects the boy and takes him on many thrilling adventures. The old king represents me and the little kid is Teddy. There's one adventure in the story he never lets me change. This is when the king and the kid look in a cave and they together discover a mushroom that when you touch it it sends beautiful fireworks all over the sky and inside the king and inside the kid, too.

But finally I did get too fed up with always telling him the same part about the cave, so one time I changed it in spite of him yelling protests at me.

I took the king and the kid off to explore the empire of the dolphins. They had to grow fins to do this exploring, then they grew scales and then they got to have whole fish bodies. And finally their skins got smooth like dolphins are. I made one of the fishes into a child-fish and the other into a king-fish. Eventually the chief dolphin conferred dolphinhood on Teddy and then on me. Teddy screamed with delight.

The empire of the dolphins is where you are safe from people rules.

Teddy indeed has lots of the symptoms of senility—won't keep his mind on anything for too long, forgets even where his feet are, hardly ever thinks of tomorrow, wants to be loved instead of being talked down to with kindness. He likes chocolate-chip cookies just as much as I do and we both absolutely can't stand beet greens.

I suppose I could get sentimental, telling you about Teddy.

The reason I'm writing about him and me is to tell you that if I hadn't been senile we wouldn't have ever gotten to be buddy-buddy. Going by the calendar, he and I are very far apart because of there being seventy years between us. Both of us are close to "the other side." The way it is with us is that we both sort of manage to get ahold of one end of the rope apiece—and then we move around so that we end up meeting face to face, and the rope gets made into a circle by the way we go with it.